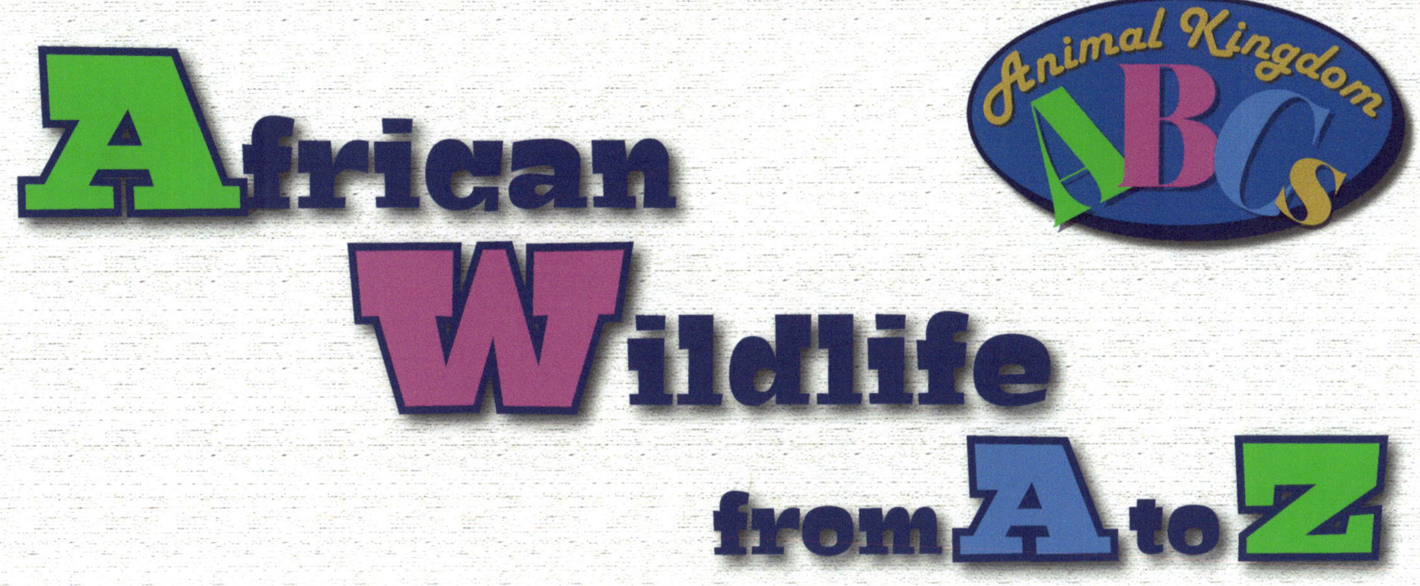

A Photo Journey Exploring the Fascinating Creatures of Africa with Fun Facts for Kids Who Love Wild Animals

by **Michele Renee Acosta**

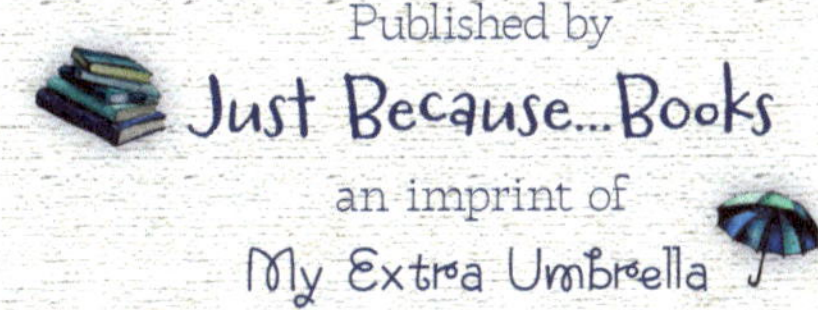

African Wildlife from A to Z:
A Photo Journey Exploring the Fascinating Creatures of Africa
with Fun Facts for Kids Who Love Wild Animals

Library of Congress Cataloging-in-Publication Data is available.
Library of Congress Control Number: 2024922753

ISBN (hardcover): 979-8-89615-061-9
ISBN (paperback): 979-8-89615-001-5
ISBN (ebook–Kindle edition): 979-8-89615-008-4
ISBN (ebook–EPUB edition): 979-8-89615-068-8

Published by
Just Because...Books
an imprint of My Extra Umbrella
1968 South Coast Highway
Suite 891
Laguna Beach, California 92651
Publisher@MyExtraUmbrella.com

This is Book 1 in the *Animal Kingdom ABCs* series.

Books in the *Animal Kingdom ABCs* series can be read in any order.

Printed in Laguna Beach, California, U.S.A.

First Edition

Author's Note

Welcome to *African Wildlife from A to Z*, a book that invites young children to embark on an exciting adventure through Africa's diverse wildlife. This book, part of the *Animal Kingdom ABCs* series, is designed to introduce children to wildlife from across the African continent in a way that's both fun and engaging. While it may look like a traditional ABC book, it goes far beyond teaching the alphabet. Instead, it's a window into the fascinating world of the animals and other wildlife that inhabit this unique part of the globe.

Each book in the series is organized alphabetically, which helps young pre-readers easily follow along and engage with the content. However, it's not about "learning the ABCs" in the usual sense. Rather, it's about sparking curiosity about wildlife and showing how vast and varied the animal kingdom can be, one letter at a time. Many of the wildlife names in this book—like *quelea* and *xenopus*—are not words typically found in a traditional ABC book. That's part of the fun! While these words may be challenging to pronounce, it's a great way for children to expand their vocabulary and learn about creatures they might never have encountered before.

Before reading for the first time, I encourage you to have a conversation about the animals children might expect to see in a book about African wildlife. Ask children to share what they already know about animals in general and African animals in particular. At the end of the book, you'll find fun facts about African wildlife, as well as critical-thinking questions designed to inspire deeper conversations. These questions are perfect for further exploration of the topic and for encouraging curiosity and a life-long love of learning.

Remember, the goal of this book is discovery and wonder. It's okay if the animal names are tricky—that's why I included helpful pronunciations and facts! This book, and the series as a whole, aims to offer children an opportunity to explore the natural world continent by continent, fostering a sense of adventure, awe, and connection to the animals with which we share this planet.

Thank you for joining me on this exciting adventure through Africa's animal kingdom!

Happy exploring!

Michele Renee Acosta

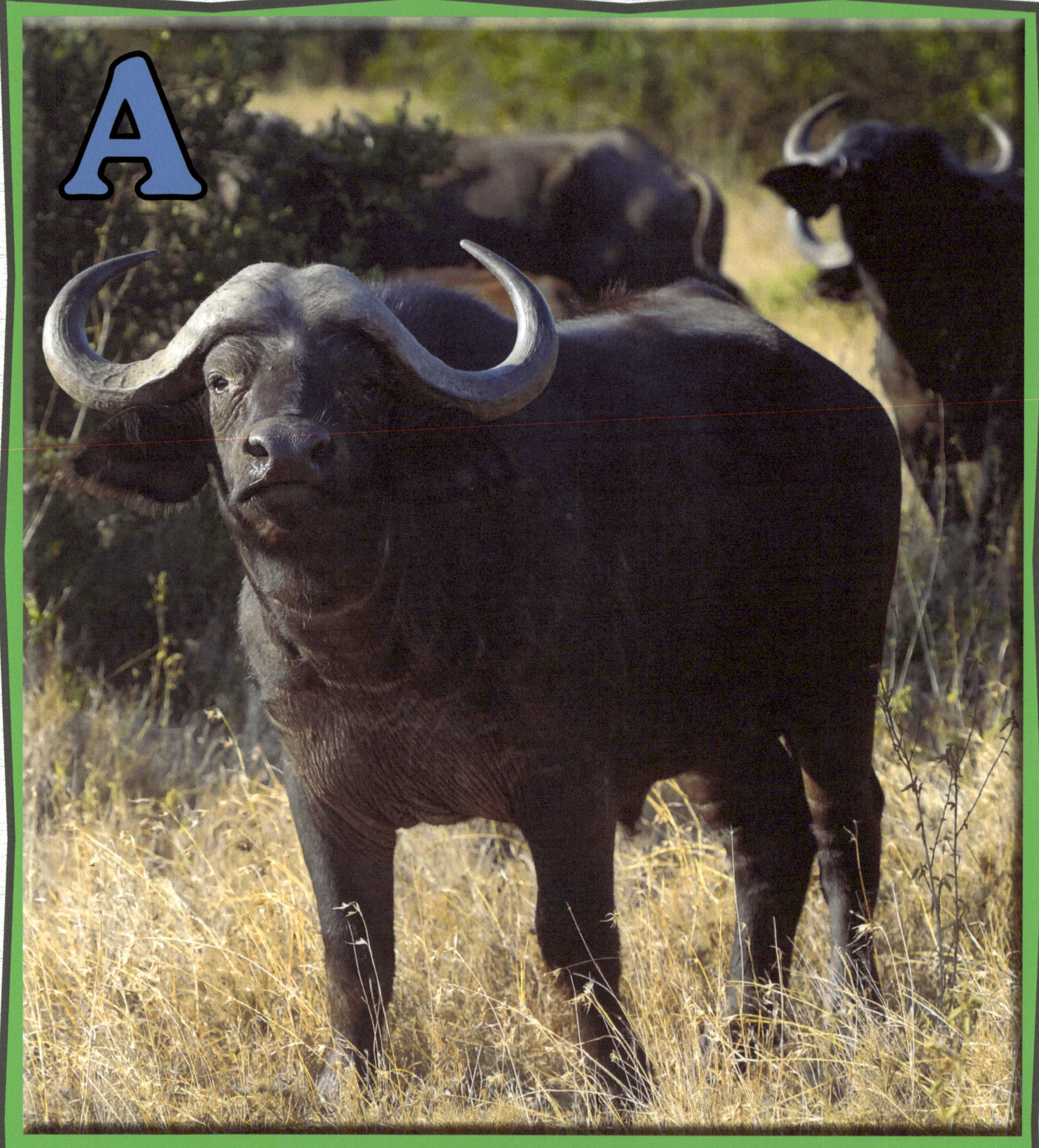

African Buffalo

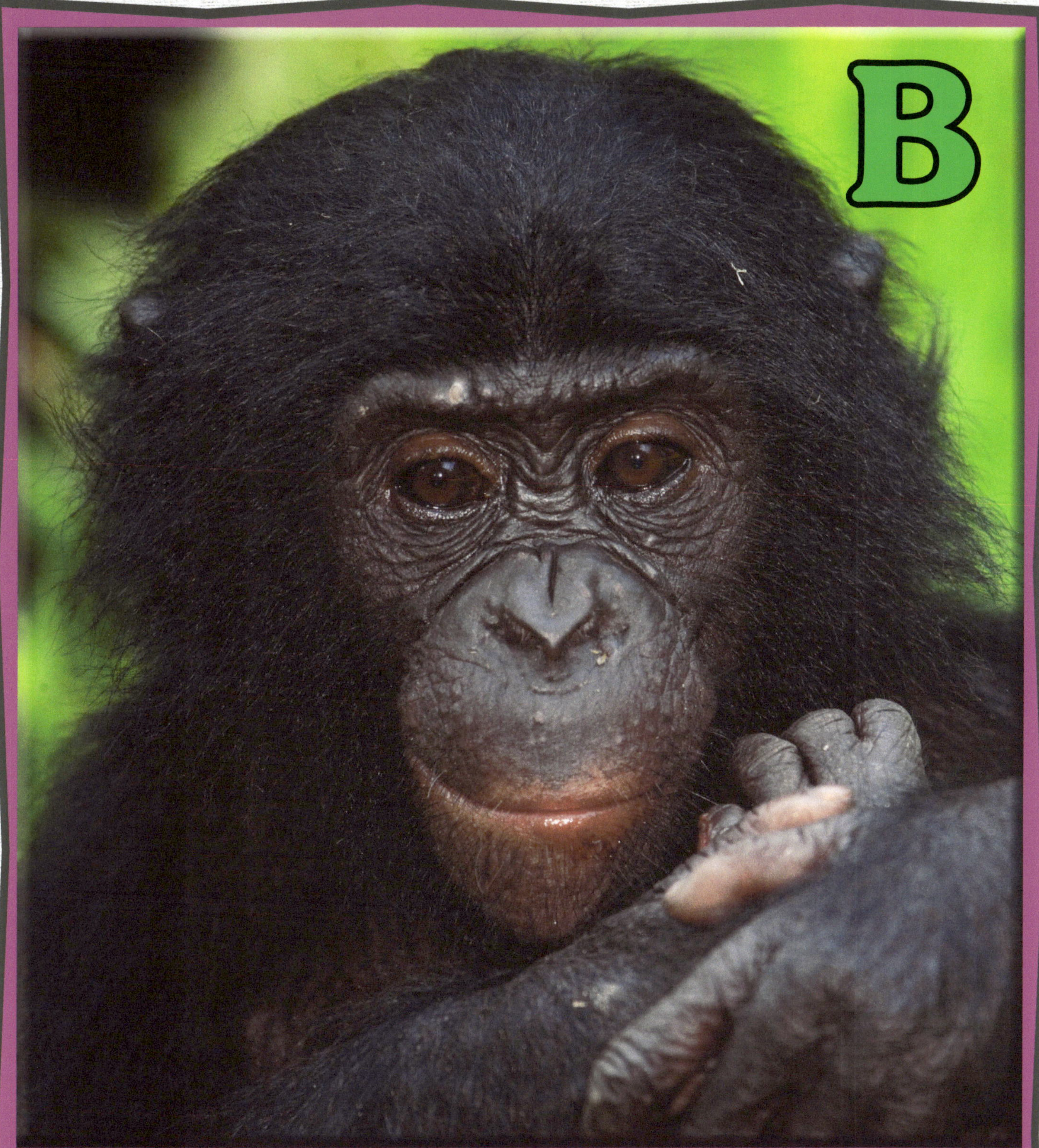

Bonobo

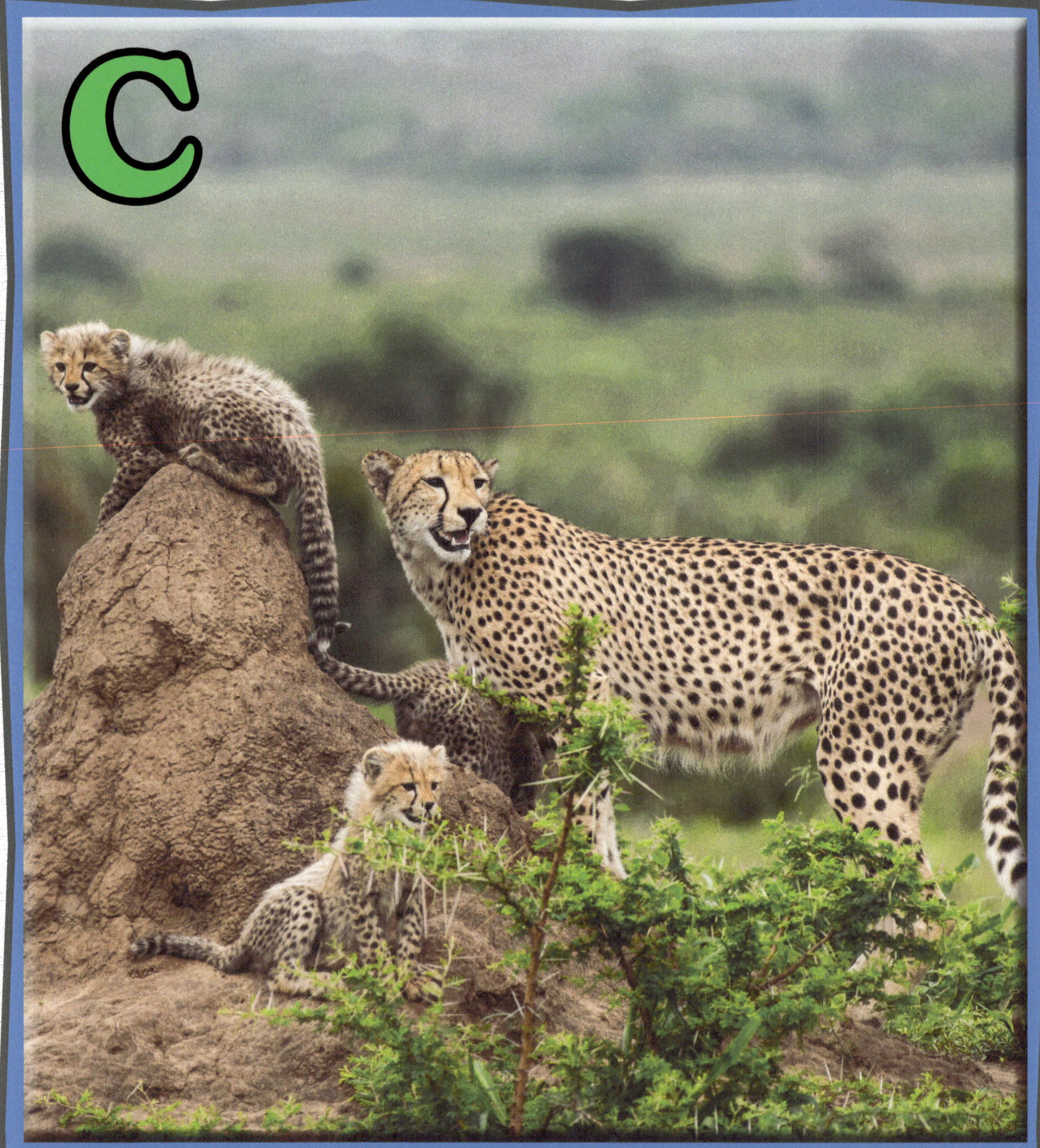

Cheetah

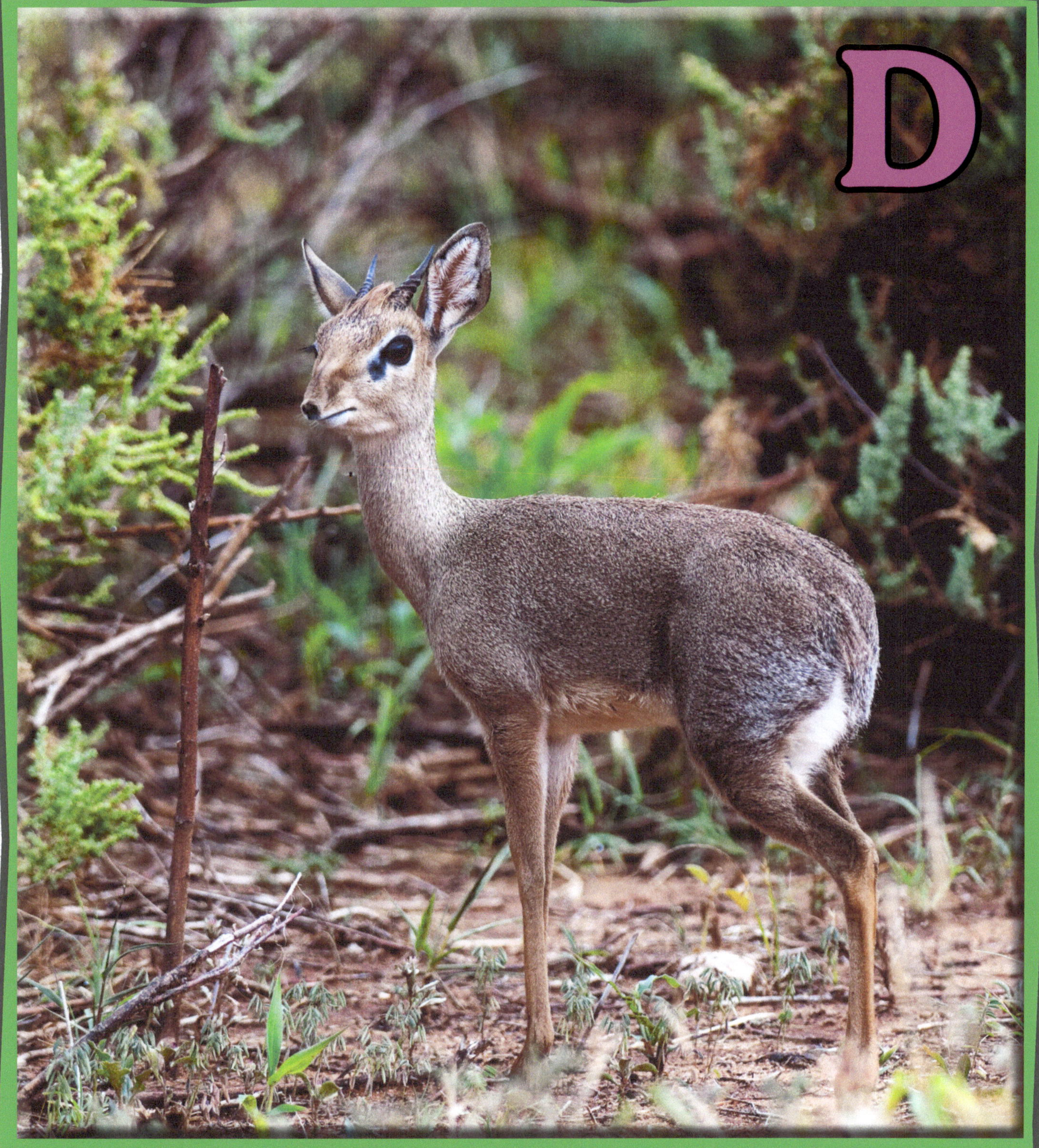

Dik-Dik

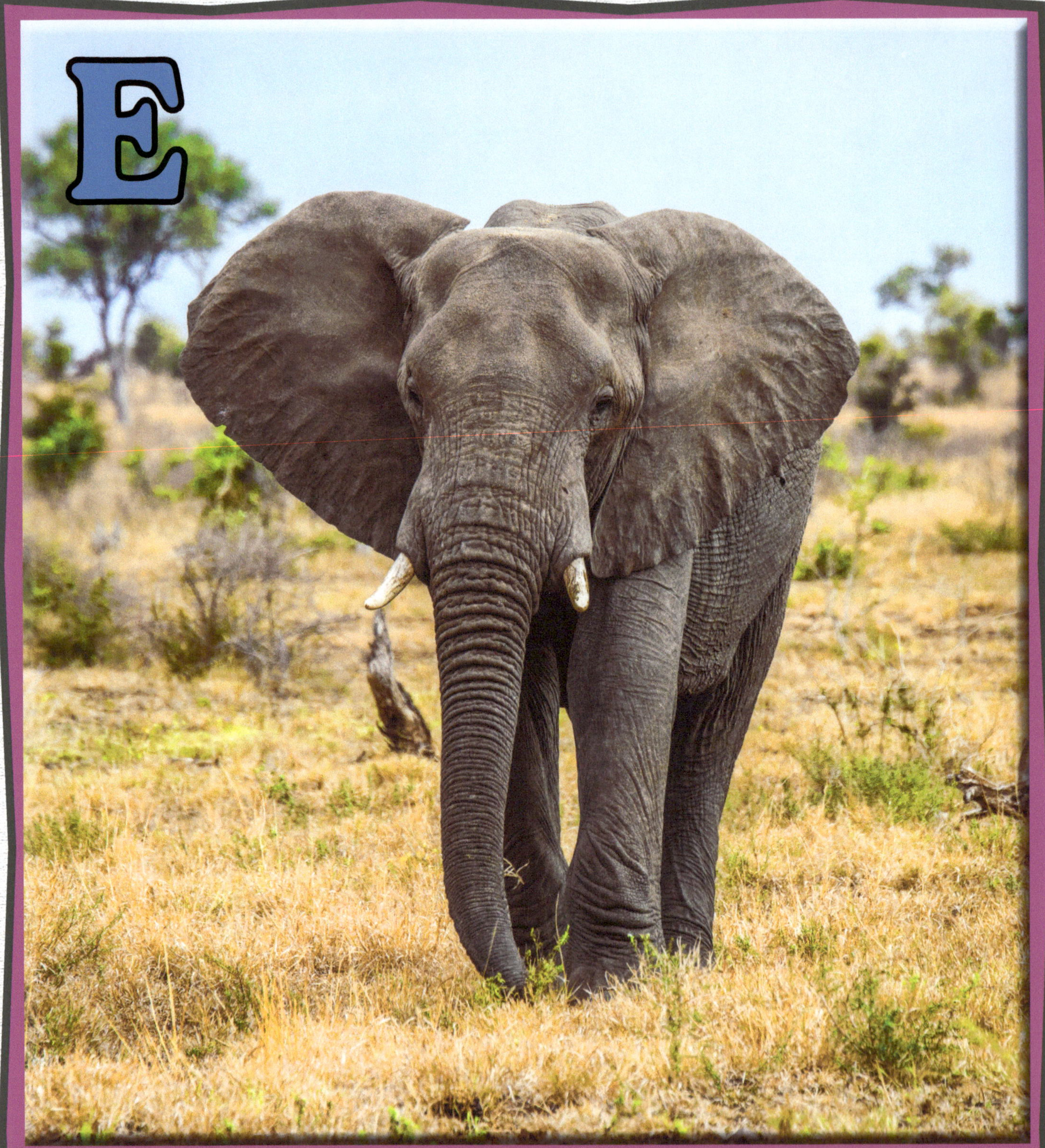

Elephant

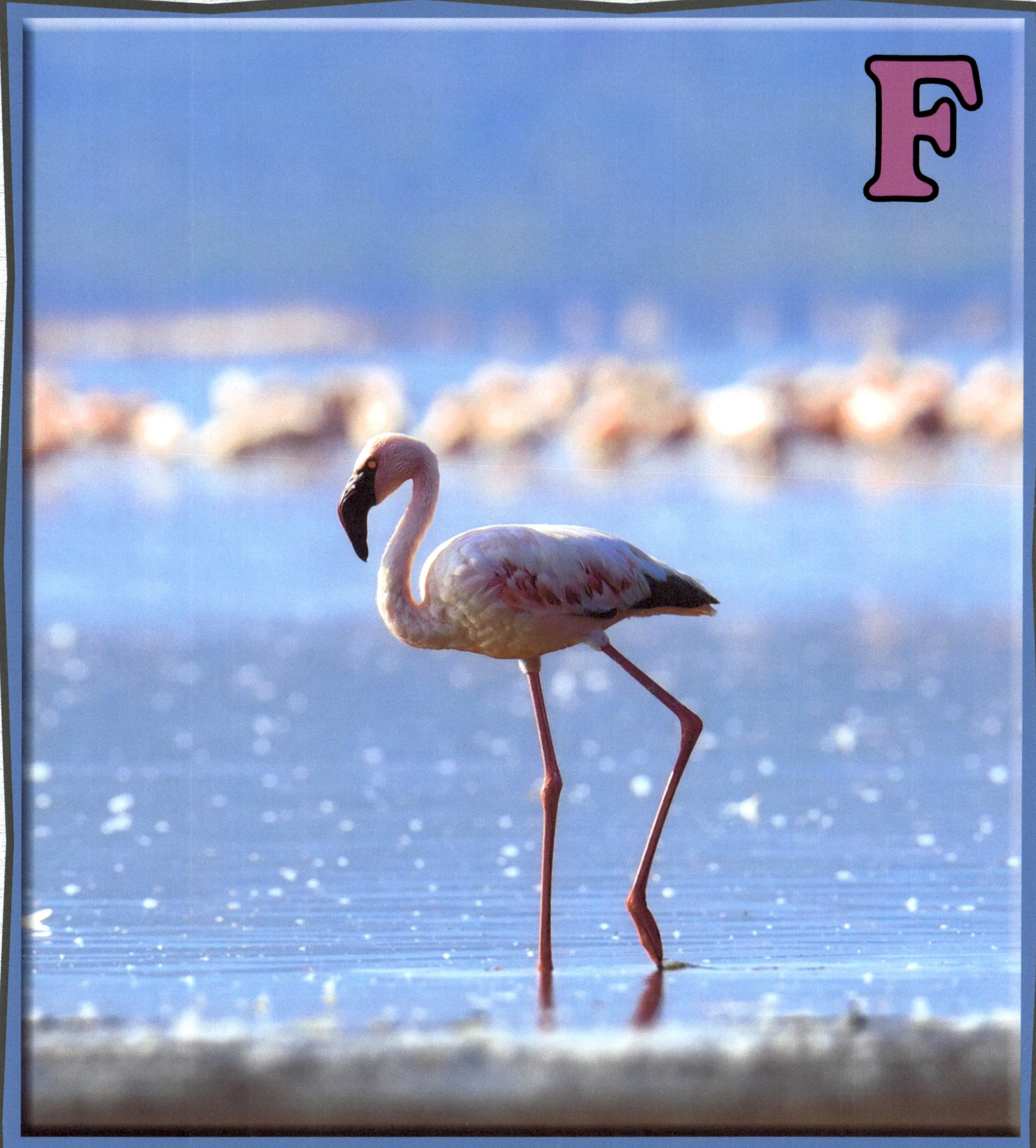

Flamingo

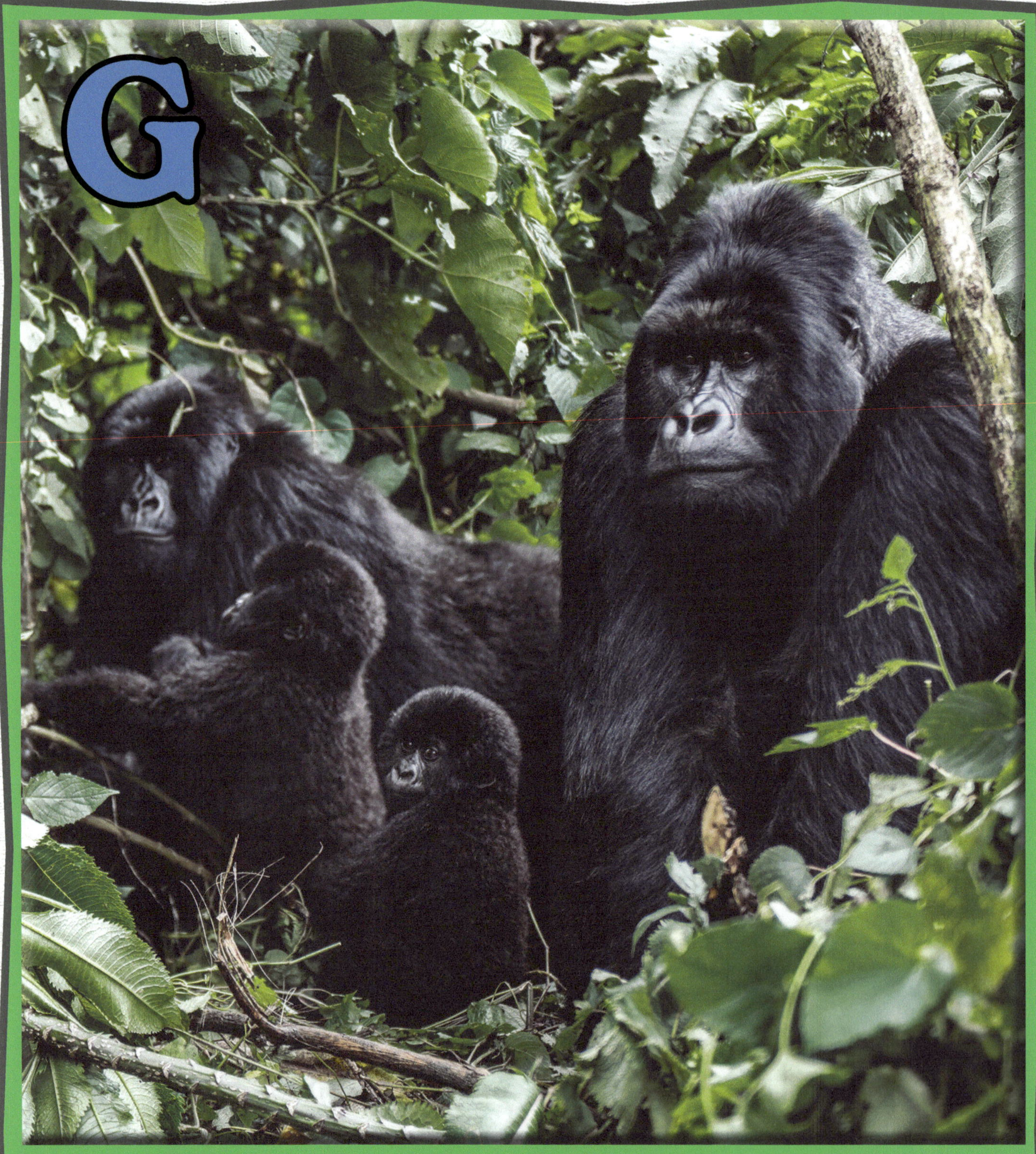

Gorilla

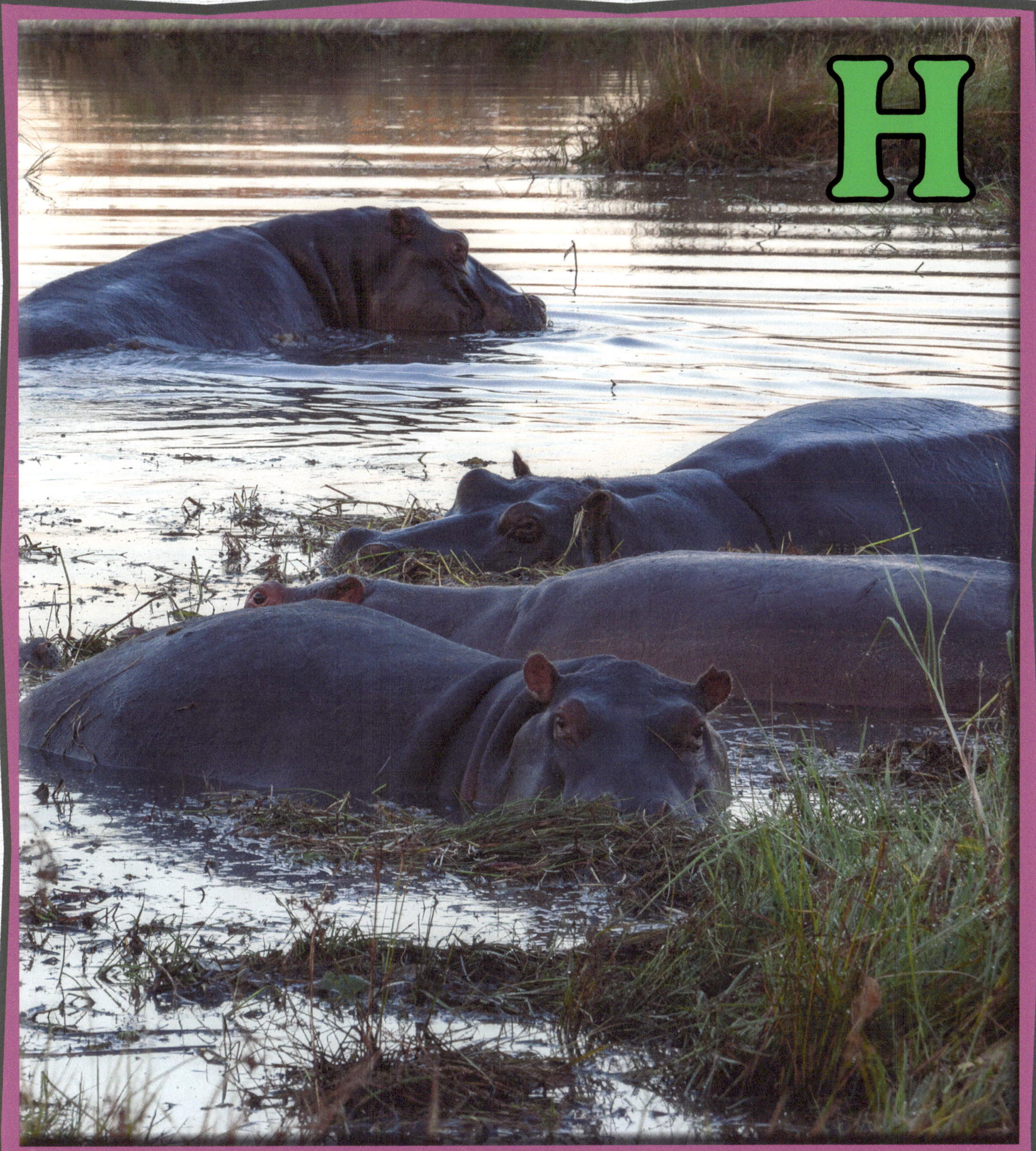

Hippopotamus

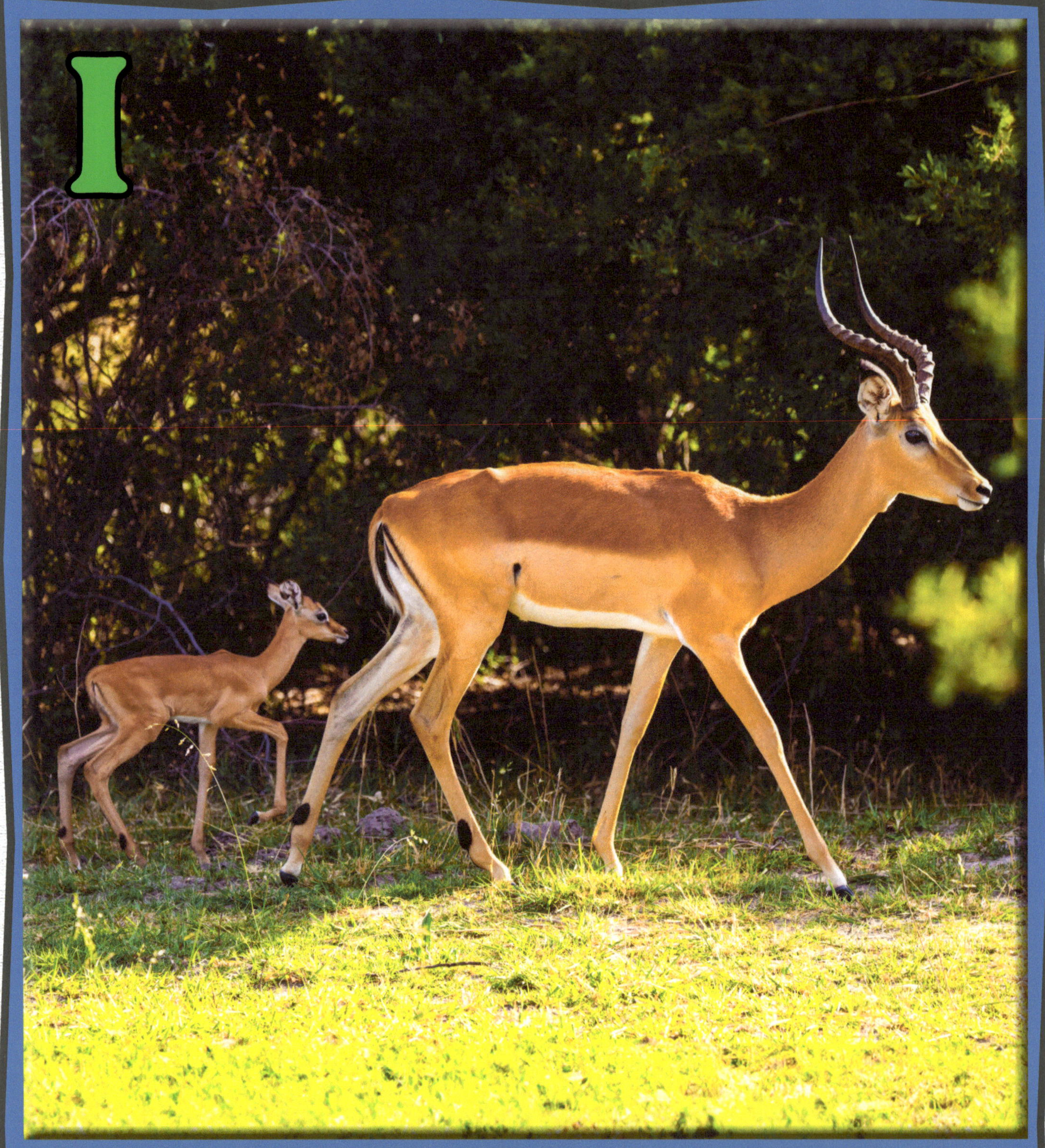

Impala

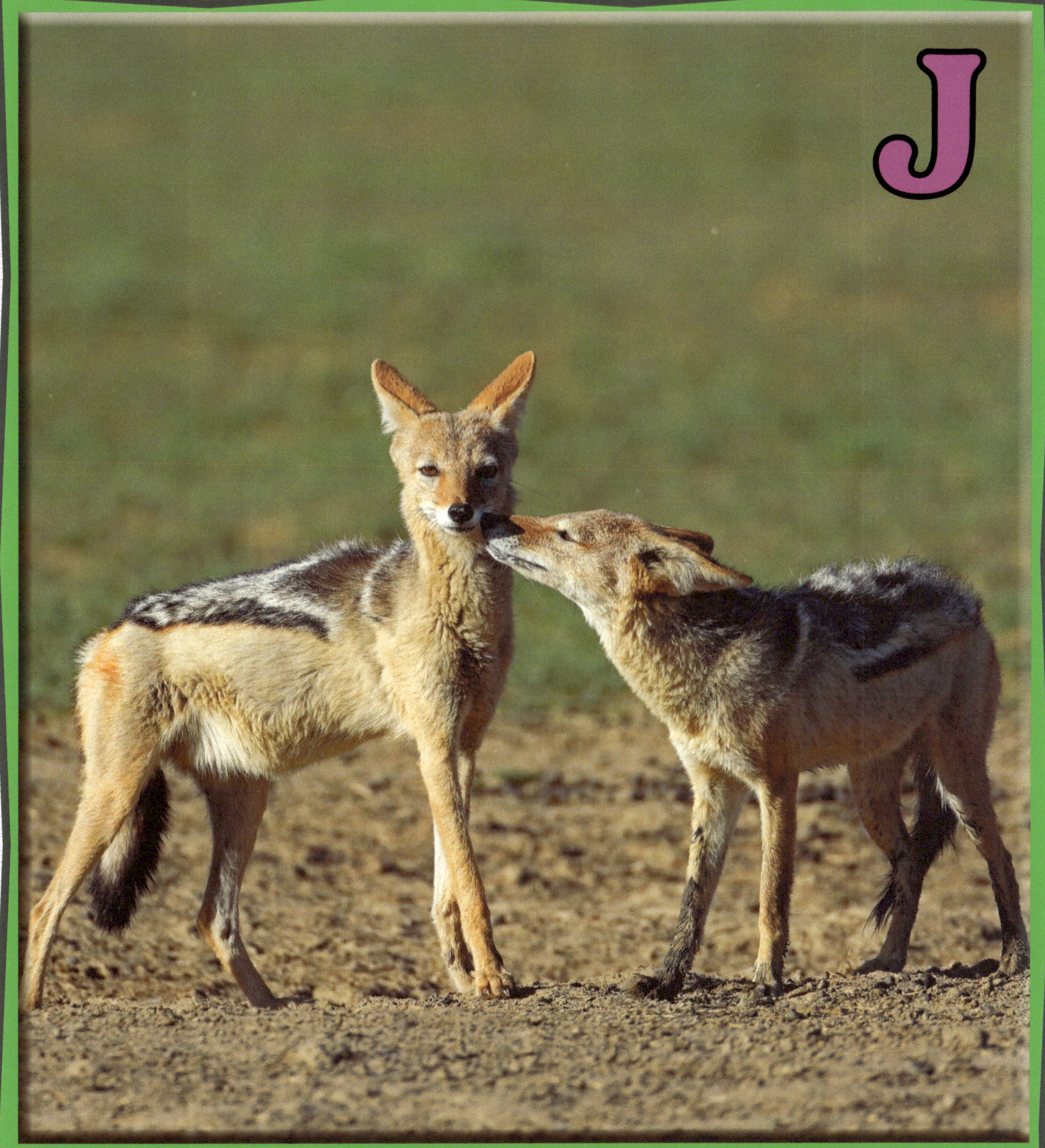

Jackal

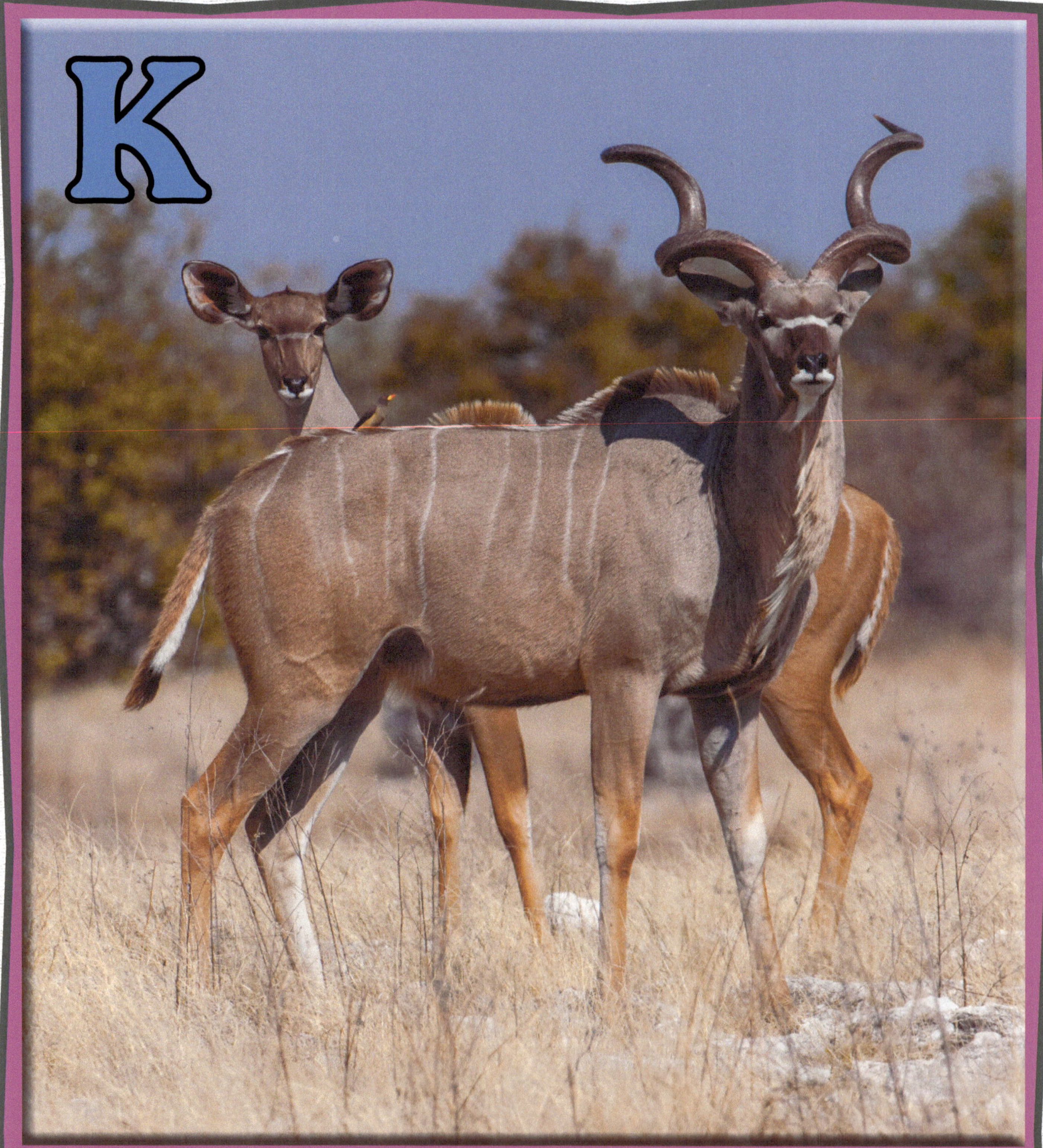

Kudu

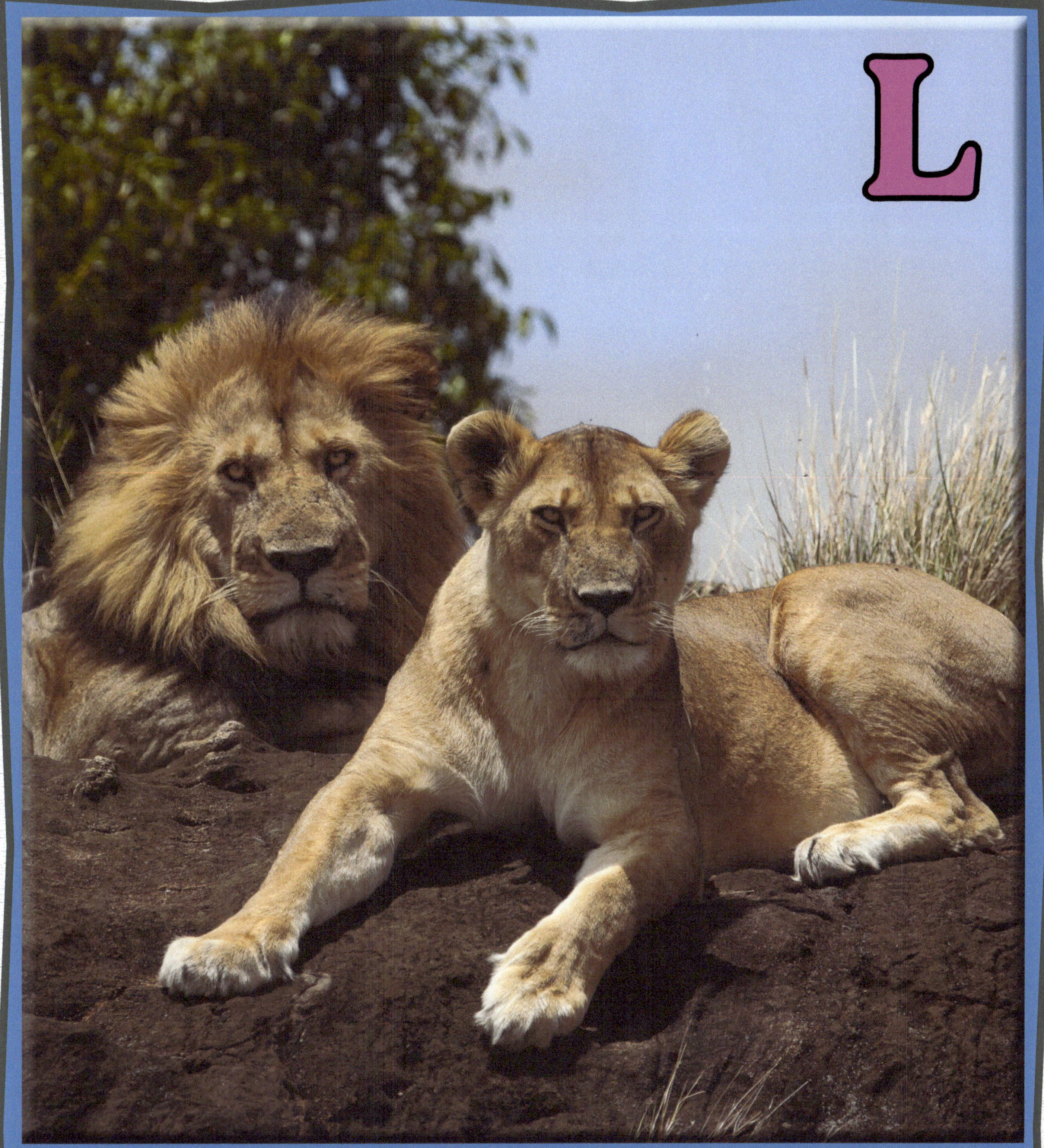

Lion

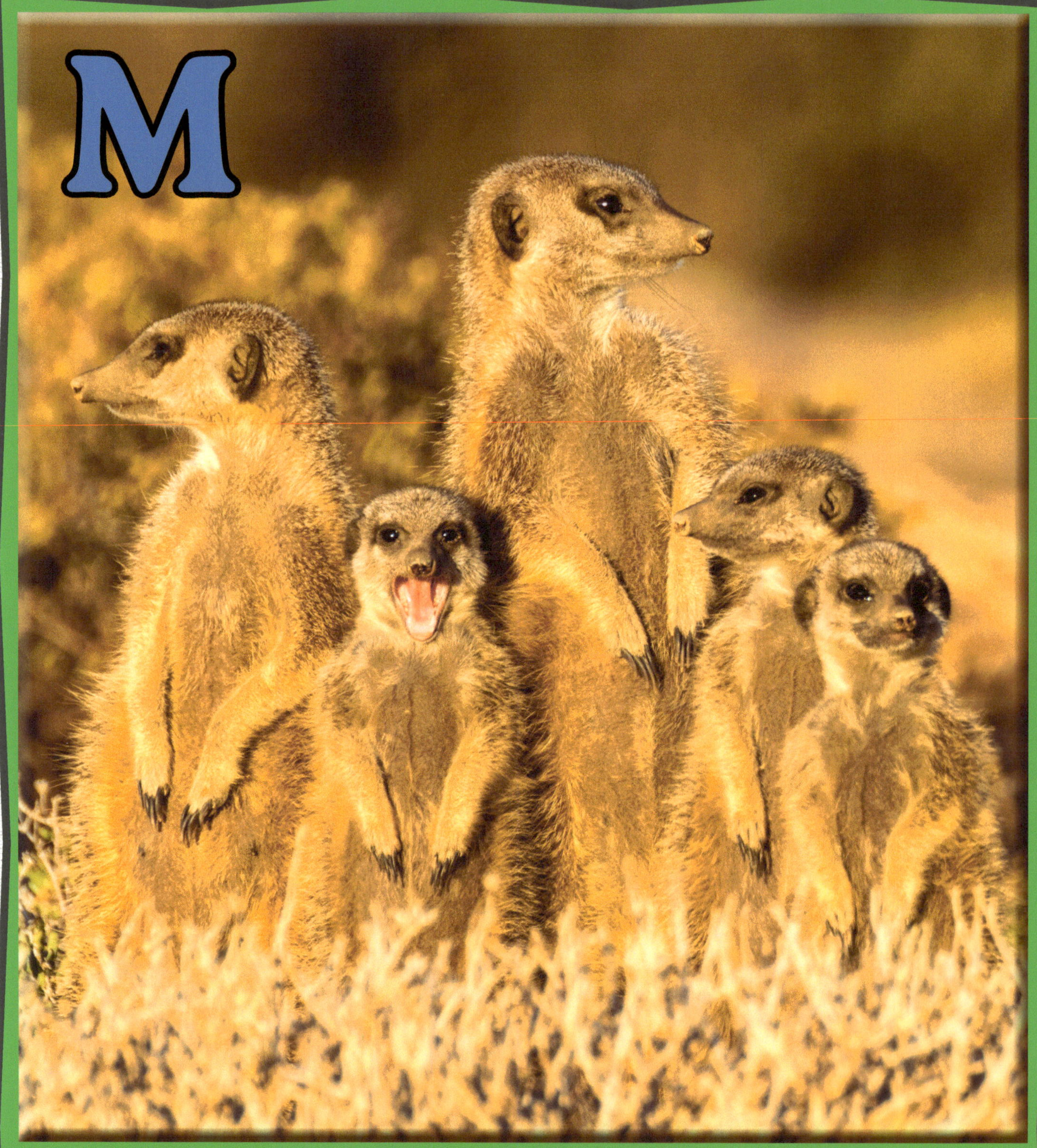

Meerkat

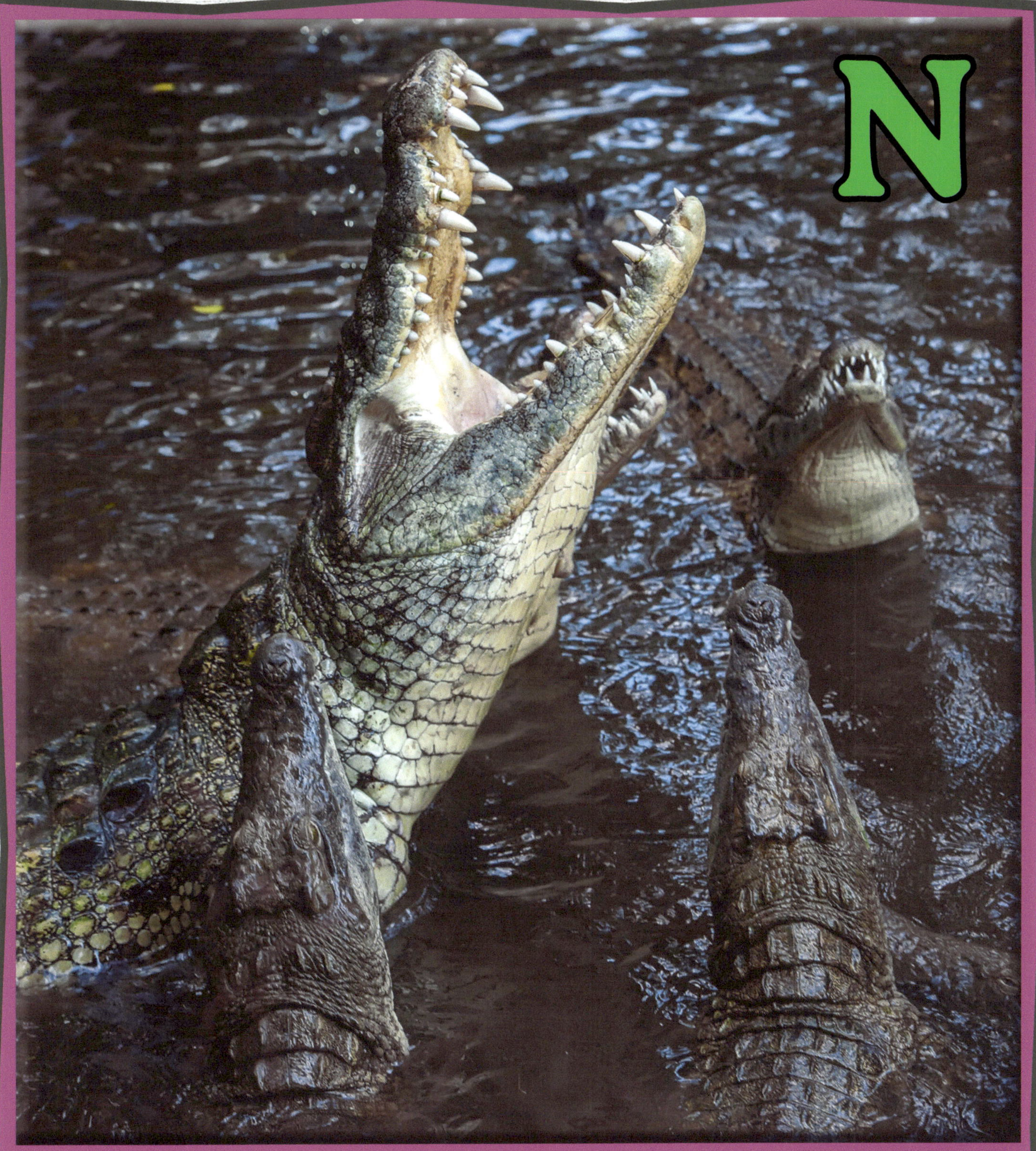

Nile Crocodile

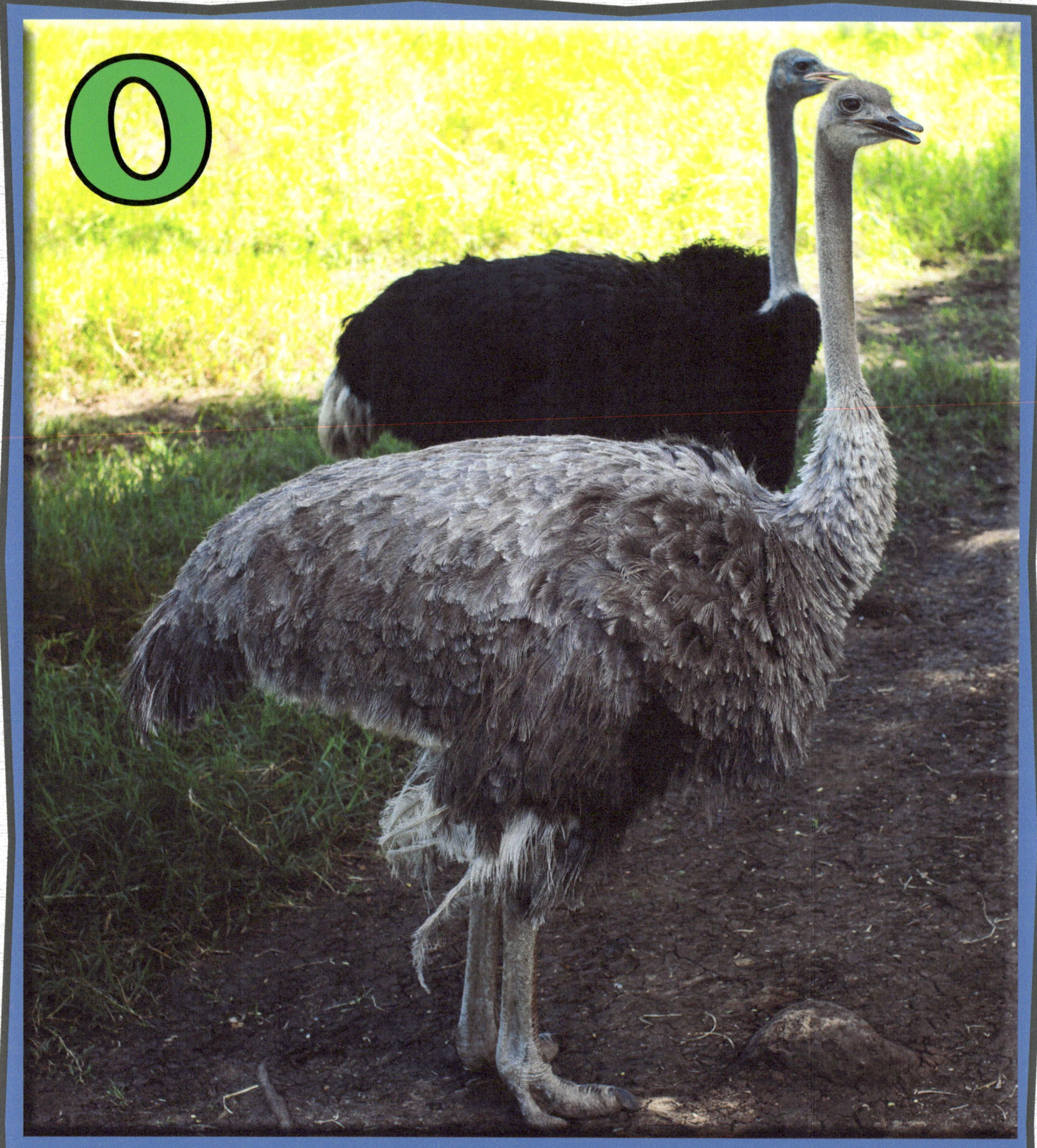

Ostrich

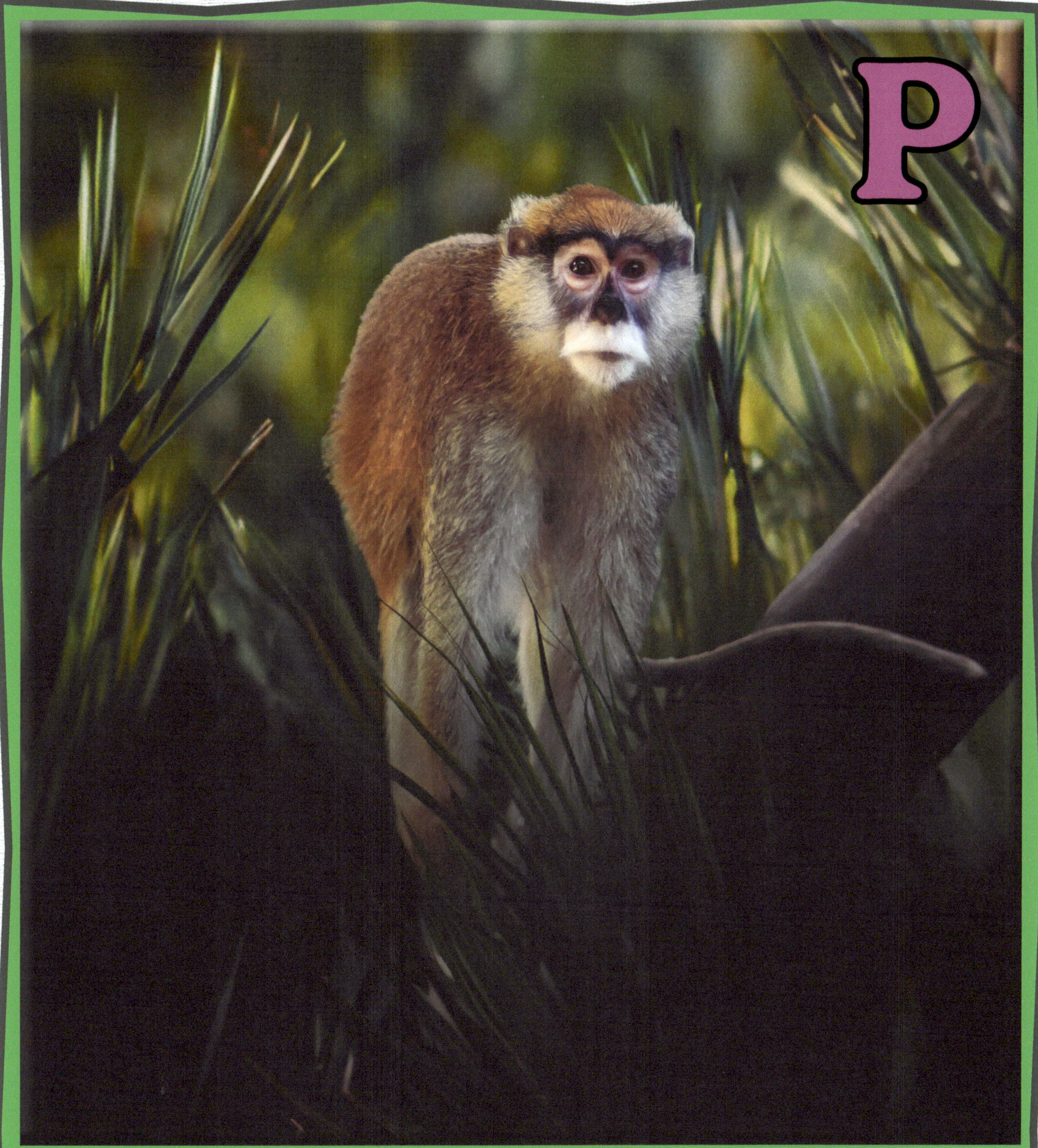

Patas Monkey

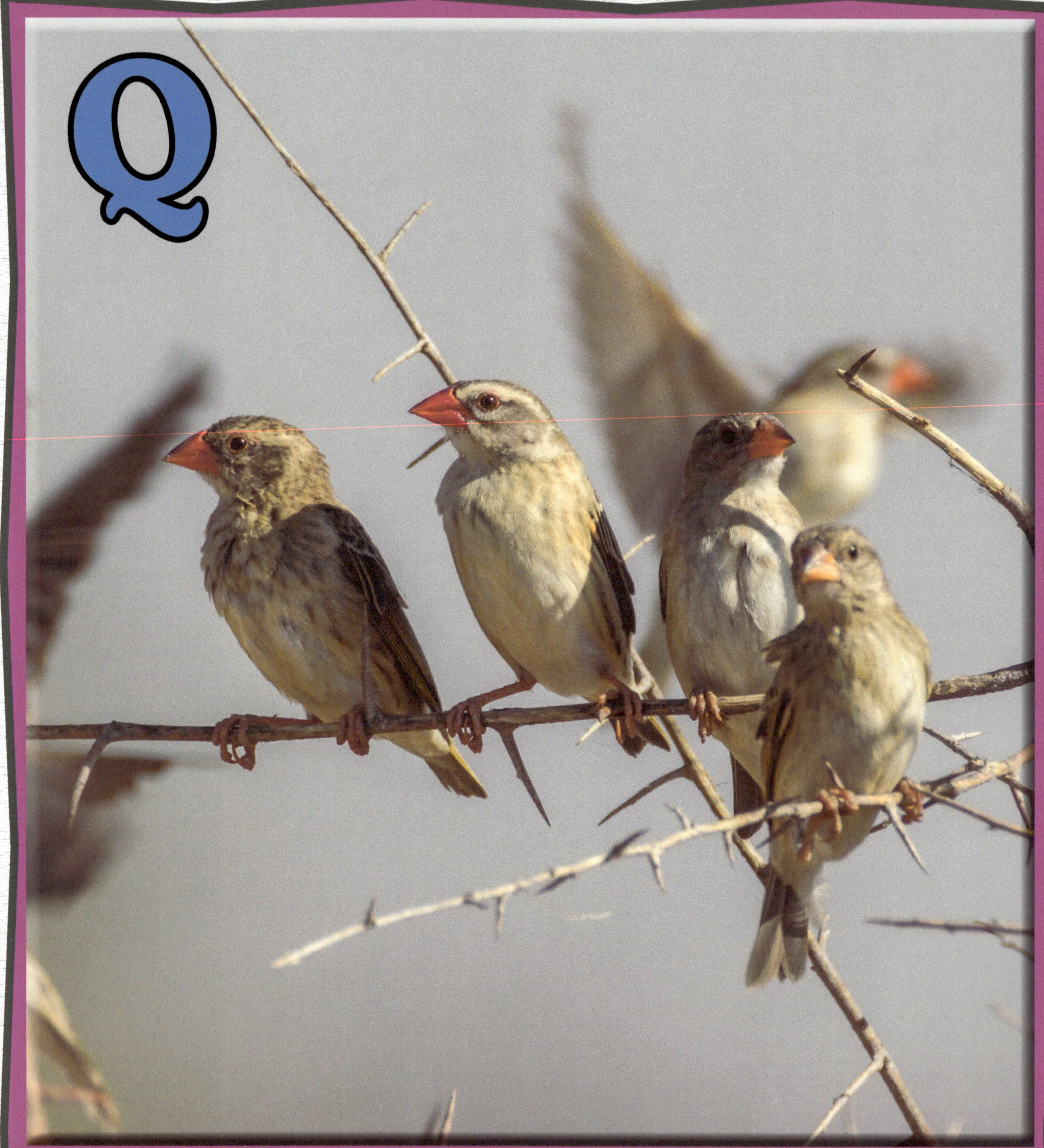

Quelea

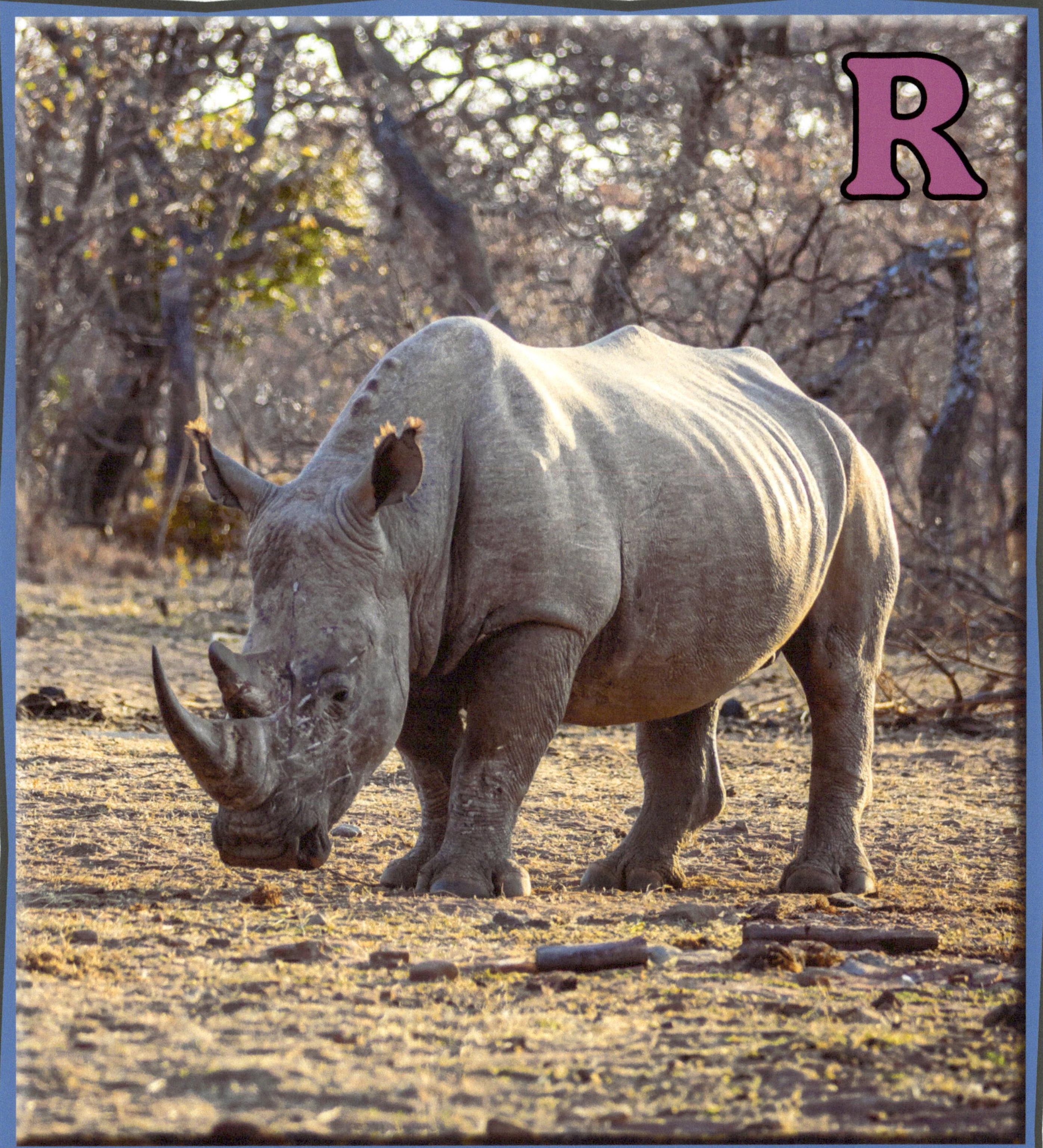

Rhinoceros

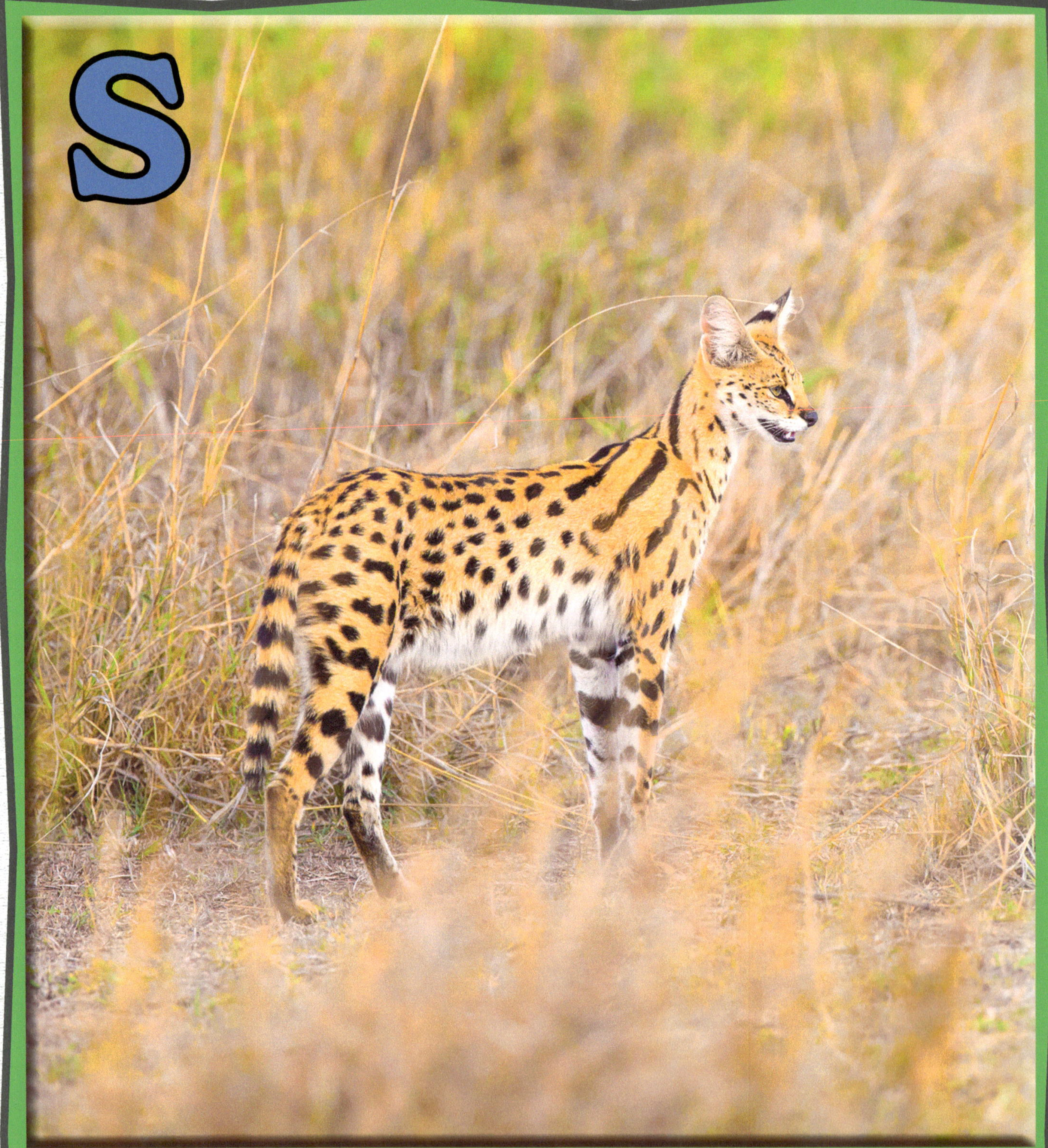

Serval

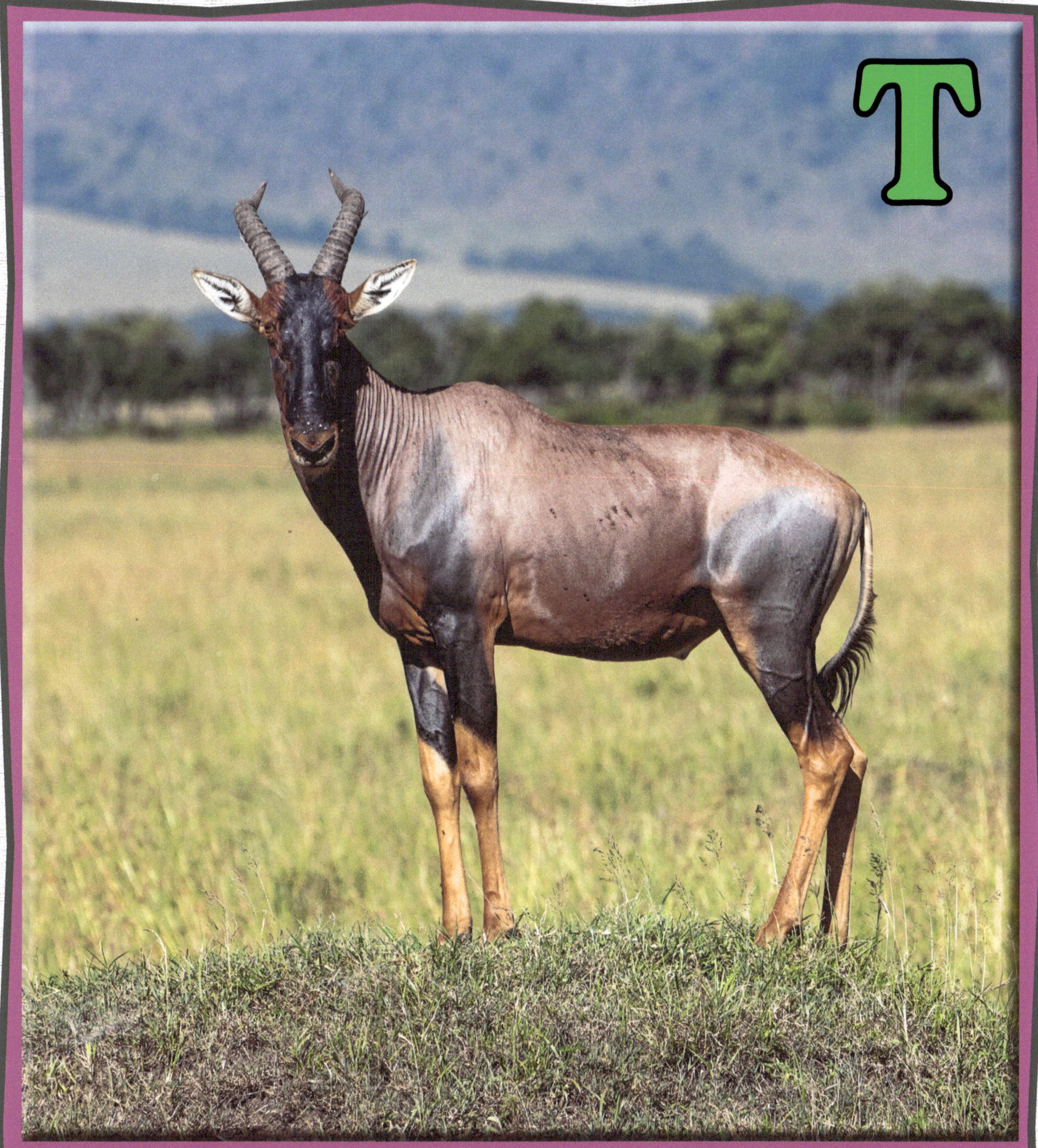

Topi

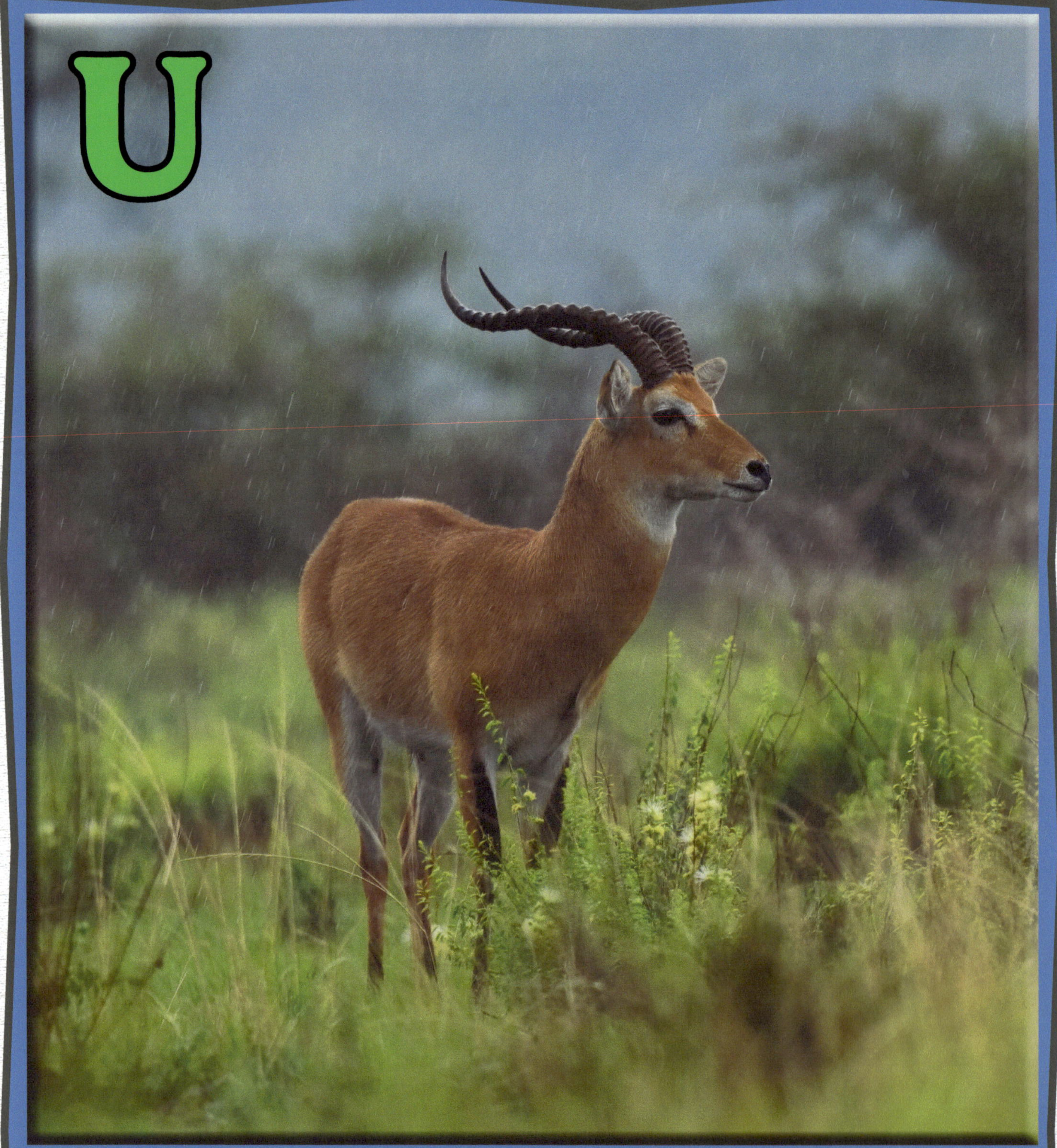

Uganda Kob

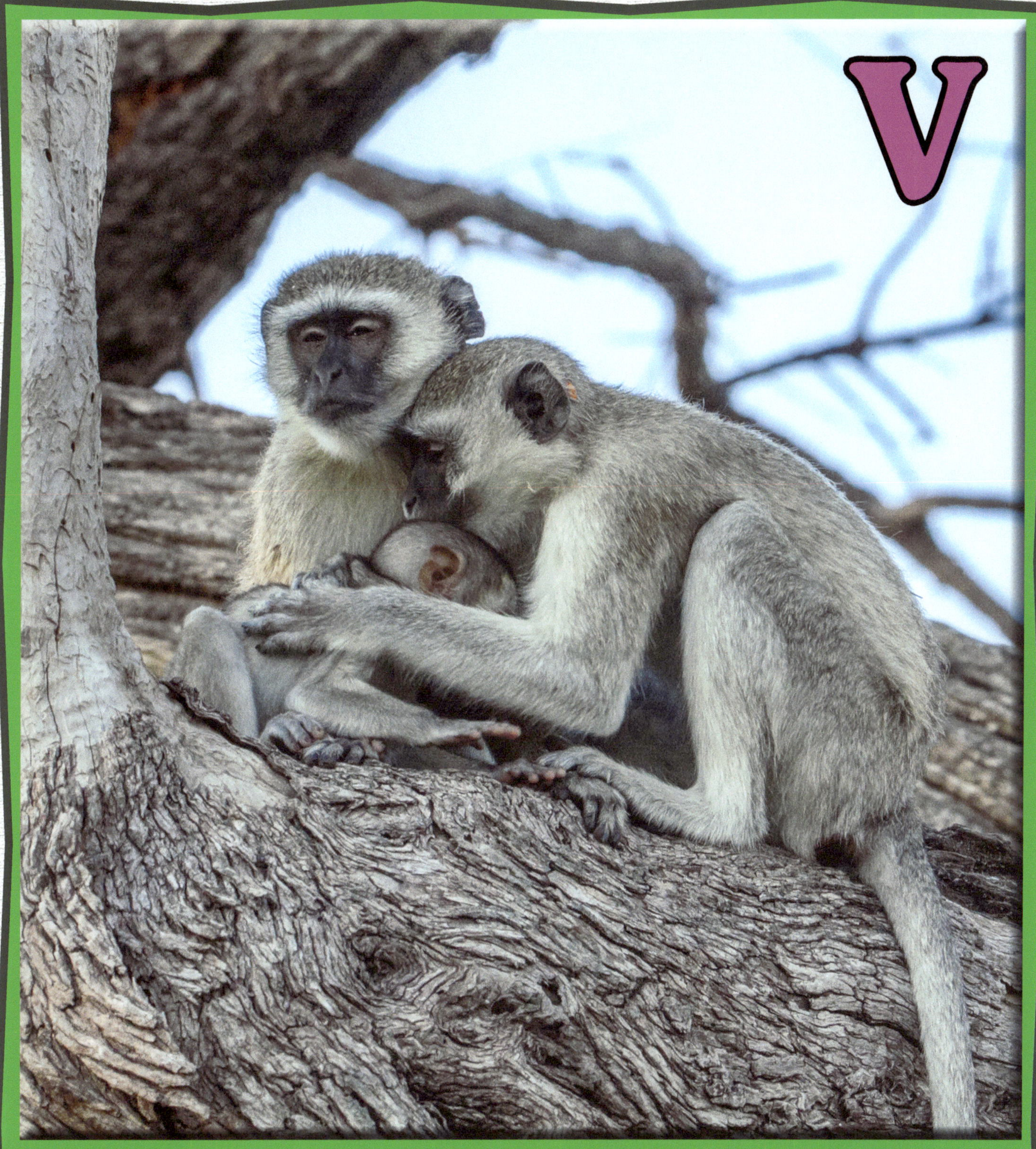

Vervet Monkey

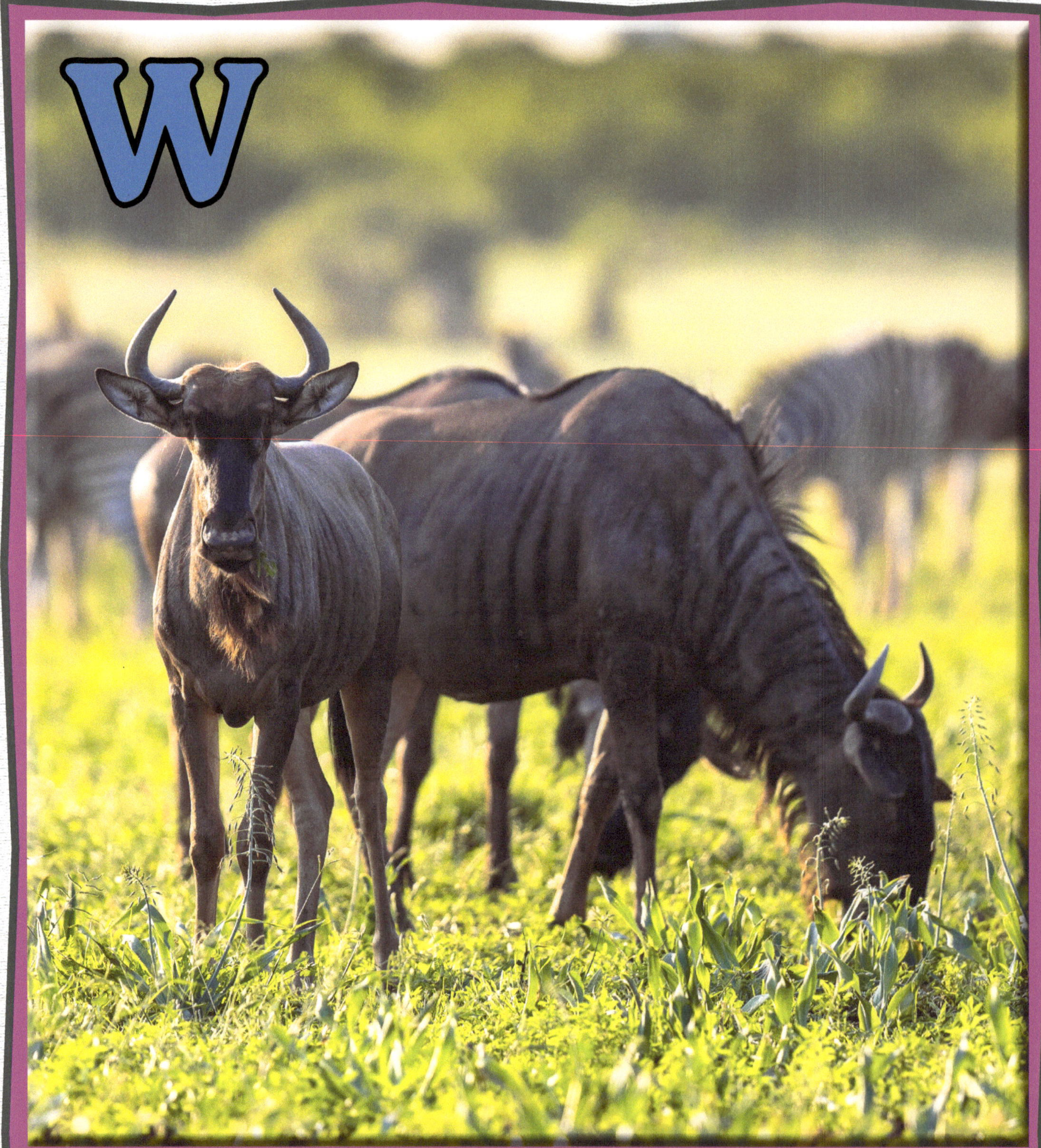

Wildebeest

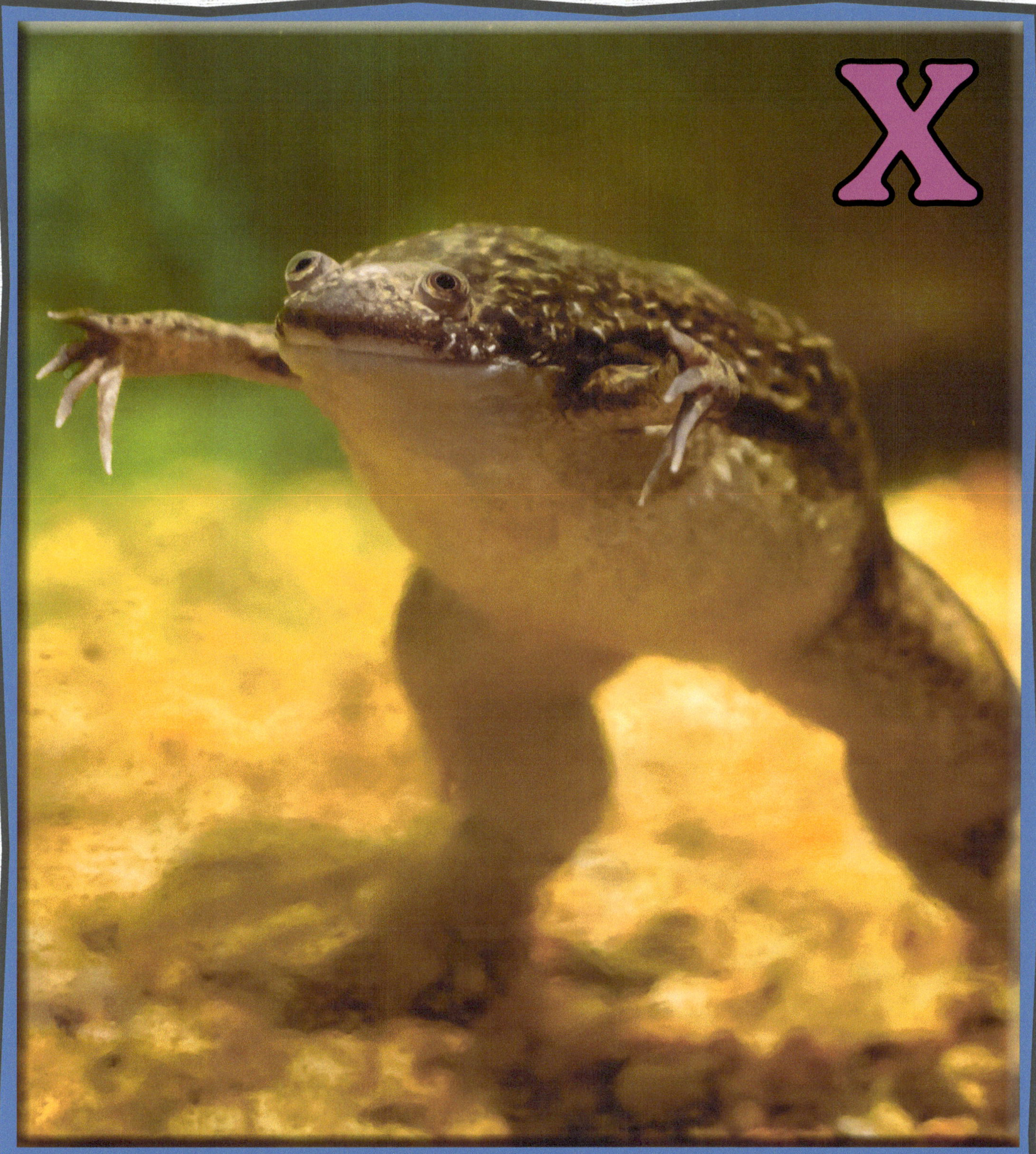

Xenopus

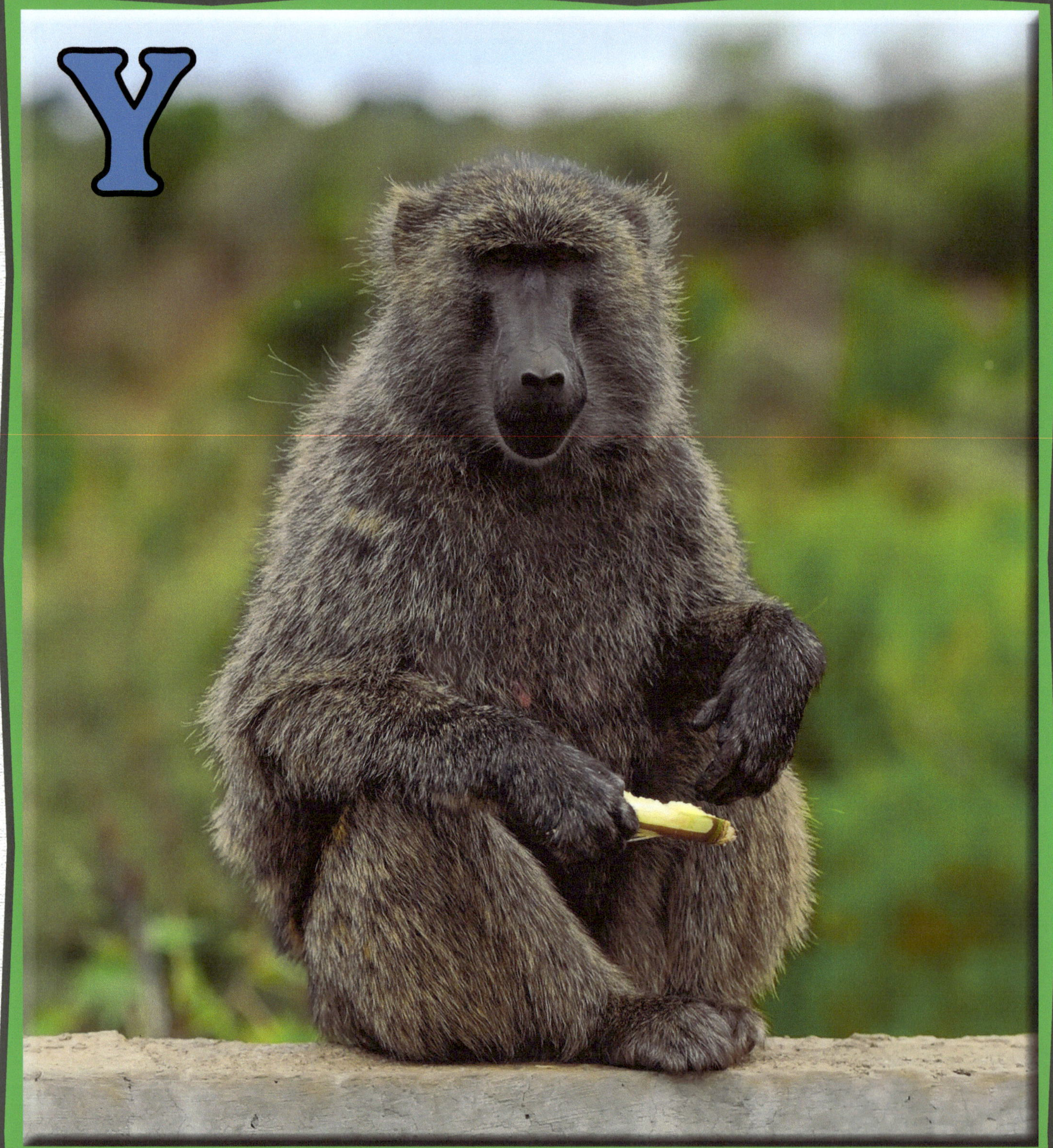

Yellow Baboon

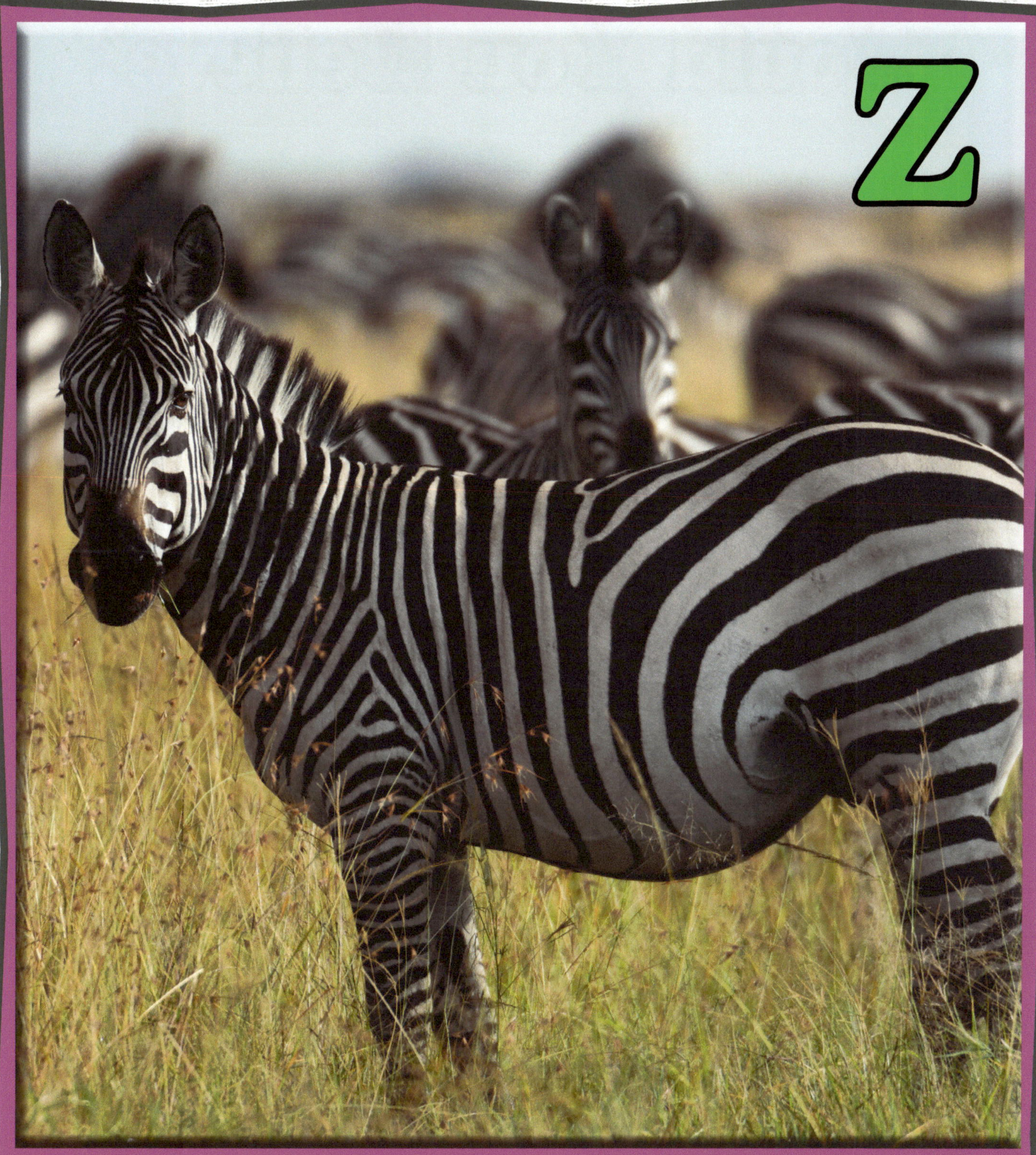

Zebra

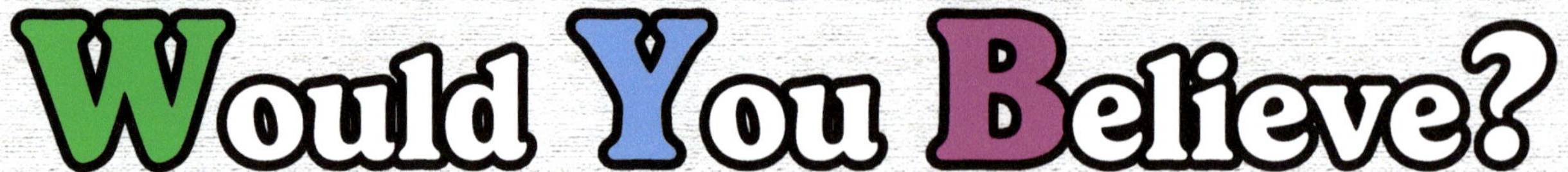

Would You Believe?

African Buffalo work together to stay safe by circling around weaker members of the herd.
Bonobos share about 98.7 percent of their DNA with humans, making them our closest living relatives.
Cheetahs don't roar! They chirp, squeak, and even purr.
Dik-Diks mark their territory using tiny scent glands near their eyes.
Elephants are among the smartest animals on Earth. They can recognize themselves in mirrors!
Flamingos turn pink because of the food they eat. They love shrimp and algae!
Gorillas build a fresh nest to sleep in every night. They build their nests on the ground or in trees.
Hippopotamuses have a natural pink "sunscreen" that helps protect their skin.
Impala can leap as far as a school bus in a single jump!
Jackals sometimes follow birds like hornbills to help find food.
Kudu have large, swiveling ears that help them hear even the faintest sounds from faraway.
Lions rest or nap most of the day—sometimes up to 20 hours!
Meerkats take turns standing guard while the others search for food.
Nile Crocodiles store fat in their tails, allowing them to go for several months without eating.
Ostriches have the biggest eyes of any animal that lives on land.
Patas Monkeys can run faster than any other monkey and as fast as a car driving 34 miles per hour!
Queleas fly together in flocks so big they can look like clouds.
Rhinoceroses skin can be almost two inches thick, but they still need to keep cool in the heat.
Servals can jump up to nine feet straight up to catch prey high in the air.
Topi climb onto little hills or mounds to watch for danger.
Uganda Kobs sometimes face each other to show who is stronger.
Vervet Monkeys have special calls to warn about different animals nearby.
Wildebeests travel 500 to 1,000 miles each year during their seasonal migrations.
Xenopus (also called African Clawed Frogs) can grow back lost body parts.
Yellow Baboons show friendship by helping each other stay clean.
Zebras have stripes as unique as human fingerprints. No two look exactly the same!

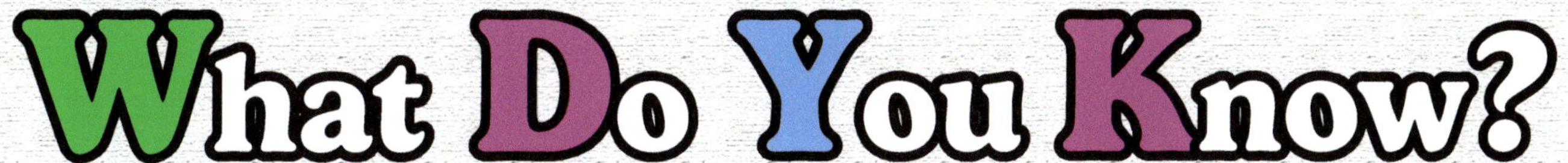

What Do You Know?

Use these questions to spark curiosity and conversation. Talk about details you notice in the photos and what you've learned together from *Would You Believe?* facts and other sources.

1. *Which African animal surprised you most? What about that animal is most interesting to you?*
2. *Which animal do you think would be easiest to spot in the wild? Which animal do you think would be hardest to spot? Why?*
3. *Which African animal would you want to see up close? Why?*
4. *How do animals like monkeys, meerkats, and African buffalo help each other stay safe?*
5. *How might big ears help an animal in the wild?*
6. *Which African animals do you think are fast runners? Which animals do you think are great jumpers? Why?*
7. *What do you think animals that live on wide open grasslands might have in common?*
8. *Which African animals do you think live in groups? Which ones might live alone? What clues helped you decide?*
9. *Pick an African animal. How do you think this animal protects itself from danger?*
10. *If you made up a new African animal, where would it live and what would it eat?*
11. *Which animals do you think make loud sounds? Which animals might make quiet sounds?*
12. *If you could be one African animal for a day, which animal would you choose? Why?*

How Do You Say It?

African Buffalo (AF-ri-kuhn BUH-fuh-loh)
Bonobo (boh-NOH-boh)
Cheetah (CHEE-tuh)
Dik-Dik (DIHK-DIHK)
Elephant (EL-uh-fuhnt)
Flamingo (fluh-MING-goh)
Gorilla (guh-RIL-uh)
Hippopotamus (HIP-uh-POT-uh-muhs)
Impala (im-PAH-luh)
Jackal (JAK-uhl)
Kudu (KOO-doo)
Lion (LY-uhn)
Meerkat (MEER-kat)
Nile Crocodile (NYL KROK-uh-dyl)
Ostrich (OS-trij)
Patas Monkey (PAH-tahs MUNG-kee)
Quelea (KWEE-lee-uh)
Rhinoceros (rye-NOS-er-uhs)
Serval (SUR-vuhl)
Topi (TOH-pee)
Uganda Kob (yoo-GAN-duh KOB)
Vervet Monkey (VUR-vit MUNG-kee)
Wildebeest (WIL-duh-beest)
Xenopus (ZEE-nuh-puhs)
Yellow Baboon (YEL-oh buh-BOON)
Zebra (ZEE-bruh)

Sources African Wildlife Foundation (https://www.awf.org); BBC Earth (https://www.bbcearth.com); National Geographic (https://www.nationalgeographic.com/animals); National Geographic Kids: National Geographic Partners (https://kids.nationalgeographic.com/animals); San Diego Zoo Kids: San Diego Zoo Wildlife Alliance (https://kids.sandiegozoo.org); Sabi Sabi Reserve: Wildlife & Nature (https://www.sabisabi.com); Smithsonian's National Zoo & Conservation Biology Institute: Animal Index (https://nationalzoo.si.edu/animals); World Wildlife Fund (https://www.worldwildlife.org/species); African Wildlife Foundation: Great Migration (https://www.awf.org)

More animals.
More fun.
More to explore.

www.ingramcontent.com/pod-product-compliance
Lightning Source LLC
Chambersburg PA
CBHW041545260326
41914CB00015B/1550
* 9 7 9 8 8 9 6 1 5 0 6 1 9 *

ISBN 0-9840839-0-1

Disclaimer

This book was written as a guide only, and does not claim to be the final definitive word on any of the subjects covered. The statements made and opinions expressed are the personal observations and assessments of the author based on his own experiences and were not intended to prejudice any party. There may be errors or omissions in this guide. As such the author or publisher does not accept any liability or responsibility for any loss or damage that may have been caused, or alleged to have been caused, through use of this information contained in this manual. The information in this book is not intended as a substitute for any exercise routine or treatment or dietary regimen that may have been prescribed by your doctor. As with all exercise and dietary programs you should get your doctor's approval before beginning. The author, editors, and publisher advise readers to take full responsibility for their safety and know their limits.

REALITY WEIGHT LOSS:

Customize, Personalize and Optimize for Simple Weight Loss Success

— — —

Tim Dutton

Your guide to creating a realistic fit, active lifestyle

TABLE OF CONTENTS

BONUS # 2: WEIGHT LOSS FUN:

INTRODUCTION

There is more information out there today, about fitness and weight loss, then there ever has been before. Yet, obesity is a major epidemic and is more of a problem in America than it ever has been in the past.

There are tons of fitness and weight loss information resources such as:

- Personal trainers
- Books and e-book's
- Internet websites
- Magazines
- Doctors
- Nutritionists
- Audio products
- Video products
- And many other various resources

Even with these resources available weight problems ranging from being slightly overweight to chronically obese is on the rise in America.

Why?

PROBLEMS OF RESOURCES

In my opinion the reason for continued obesity is that the information out there has various problems. Below is a list of what I believe to be the most common problems.

Information overload

Most of the information products out there list too much unnecessary information. The average person cannot sort through this to gain usable information. Most of the information resources available, go overboard with scientific jargon and terms. Too much information can be just as bad, as not enough information. There should be a balance developed between enough information and too much information. You do not have to have a college education or be a rocket scientist in order to lose weight.

Over complicated

A lot of the so-called "experts" operate under what I like to refer to as ego-based instruction. These "experts" are more interested in having people believe that they are extremely intelligent, rather than being concerned with how much they are helping people. Fitness and weight loss is not rocket science. The simpler it is, the easier it is going to be for you to start and maintain.

One-size-fits-all systems

People are bombarded with loads of prearranged workouts and diets. In reality every individual is different with different needs, wants, desires, problems, goals, etc. For a workout to truly benefit each person it has to be customized to fit that persons needs.

Conflicting information

A lot of the "experts" are saying that if you do not do it my way, you're doing it wrong and if you fail, it is your own fault. It seems that no two "experts" agree on how it actually should be done. In reality there is multiple ways to do almost everything, just because one way is different than another does not make it wrong. You need to find the best way that works for you.

Too much too soon

Most "experts" are more than willing to tell you where you *should* be, on eating and exercising. Unfortunately, very few show you realistic ways of getting there. It is unrealistic to expect someone to go from eating very unhealthy foods and being inactive to waking up one morning and eating completely clean and doing high intensity exercises for the rest of their life. Activity and dietary changes must be incorporated moderately with realistic goals.

Too specific

There is a ton of information out there if you are a bodybuilder, fitness model and even a mixed martial arts athlete. This is fine if you're a bodybuilder, fitness model or mixed martial artist, but what if you're not either one of these? Anytime you start to apply specific exercises, techniques or principles it should be specific to your individual needs and goals. For general health and fitness you can stick with General exercises, techniques and principles. Only start applying specifics when you determine you have specific needs or goals.

So-called functional training

There is a new term that every "expert" seems to like to throw around it is "functional training". Functional training is very beneficial, the problem lies in the perception of what is functional. What is functional for one person may not be functional for another. Functional training is the implementation of exercises that mimics functional activity within your daily life. A lot of "experts" like to claim that the bench-press is functional. I don't know about you but whether it be in my daily life or my career I have never had to lay down and do bench presses in order to complete the task. As I stated earlier functional training is very beneficial, just make sure that it is functional for you.

Boomerang dependency

What I mean by this is that a lot of products and services are designed to get you to depend on more products and services and keep you coming back. In order for you to lose weight and maintain this weight, you're going to have to take control and become self-reliant and self-sufficient. There is a lot of products and services that can be very beneficial, but keep in mind that they should be supplemental and not an absolute necessity. You possess all the necessary skills and abilities to take control of your life and your weight.

Fad diets

Extreme dietary restrictions cannot be maintained for extended periods. A lot of people get the ideal that they will be able to follow one of these fad diets, until they lose weight, and then return to eating as normal. Problem is if they return to eating like they was before, they are going to regain the lost weight, and possibly more because of a slowed metabolism. In reality, whatever you do to lose weight will most likely be what you have to continue to do in order to maintain the weight loss. Therefore any dietary changes should be ones you can realistically maintain for the rest of your life.

Magic pills

A lot of companies want to sell you their very own, newly discovered magic weight loss pill or exercise in a bottle. If there actually was a magic pill, we would not have the weight problems we have today. The only true and safe way to control weight is through diet and exercise. Keep in mind that supplements are just that, *supplements* to exercise and diet's, and should be used with caution and not abused.

Biased opinions

Traditional bodybuilders claim you must work out with weights for high volume of sets. High intensity bodybuilders claim you must work out with weights to absolute failure for one set. Pilates and yoga participants claim all you need is your body and coordination of breathing. Marathon runners believe you must run long distances to be fit and healthy. There is a multitude of various groups that believe in different styles of training. So who's right? All and none of them are right, as we mentioned earlier there is multiple right ways to train and multiple right types of equipment. All are beneficial to some degree, and will have their own unique pros and cons, you must decide which one is right for you.

These are In my opinion some of the most common problems but definitely not all. Let's see if we can correct some of these problems.

ABOUT THIS BOOK

Before we get started I'd like to give you a little bit of information about this book such as: why I wrote it, who it's for, what this book is and what it is not.

WHY I WROTE THIS BOOK

There is various reasons why I wrote this book. The primary reasons I wrote this book are as follows:

Personal consumer disappointments

I have personally purchased and used various products and systems to no avail. Nothing seemed to work, and everything out there seemed to be targeted toward everyone but me. I am not a bodybuilder, I am not a professional athlete and I am definitely not a fitness model. I am a private investigator, a bounty hunter, a concrete finisher, a self- defense instructor and even at times a personal trainer, but most importantly I am a person who wants to have a healthy weight for everyday purposes. I would always be excited whenever I started something new, sometimes I would start to see results, but ultimately in the end I was disappointed and right back where I started.

Certified personal trainer

As you can see above, I mentioned that I'm a personal trainer. I've actually been certified through several different organizations. My current certification is as a N.E.S.T.A. (National Endurance and Sports Trainers Association) certified advanced personal trainer. Therefore I believe I have the basic knowledge and understanding for fitness and weight loss to give you sound and effective principles for controlling your weight.

Commonsense approach

I also wrote this book because I wanted to give you principles and advice based on common sense. Common sense is something that, today seems to not be very common. I believe that common sense will take you farther and allow you to achieve goals more easily, than any other of the so-called scientific and expert opinions.

Non-ego-based opinions

As you've probably noticed, I do not hold a great deal of respect for the term "expert". In my experience, once most people perceive themselves to be experts, they believe they know everything there is to know about a subject, and close their mind and stop learning. I never have and never will consider myself an expert, therefore I always keep an open mind and try to learn something every day.

Personal experience

One other reason I wrote this book is experience. I'm not talking about the 22 years I've spent learning and training about fitness. I am talking about experience with weight problems. Including perceived weight problems all through high school, and actual weight problems for several years after high school. I believe that someone who has never experienced weight problems, cannot truly understand what someone with weight problems goes through.

That is some of the reasons I wrote this book, but in short I wrote this book to help people who are experiencing weight problems like I did.

Now let's move on and discuss.....

WHO THIS BOOK IS WRITTEN FOR

I believe this book will benefit a great number of people, however as there was primary reasons I wrote this book, there is also primary groups of people I wrote this book for. Following are the primary groups of people I wrote this book for.

People who want to simplify

The simpler a program is, the easier it will be to stick with and maintain for extended periods of time. Therefore I wrote this book for people who want to simplify weight loss, weight maintenance and overall weight control.

People who want to take control

Most people who are overweight feel their lives are out of control, in order to lose weight you must gain control. Therefore this book is also written for people who want to take control of their weight and life, and who want to stop feeling like their life is spiraling out of control.

People who want to customize

The best weight-loss method or system is one that is customized and personalized to fit your lifestyle. So this book is written for people who want to customize their dietary habits and exercise activities to fit their own personal goals and lifestyles.

People who want a realistic approach

In order to effectively lose weight and maintain the weight you must use realistic methods and apply common sense. Therefore this book is written for people who want realistic weight control methods that utilizes common sense, that they can maintain for the rest of their life.

People who are fed up with fad diets

As we mentioned earlier in order for weight loss to be most efficient you must simplify and customize. Fad diets and gimmicky programs will only set you up for failure, they are usually unrealistic and cannot be maintained for prolonged periods of time. So the last group of people that this book was written for, are people who are tired of trying and failing on fad diets and gimmicky exercise routines.

In short, if any part of this list applies to you, then this book is written for *You*.

WHAT THIS BOOK IS

This book is a guide that was designed to be easily read and understood, it is designed to help you do the following things:

Simplify

This book is designed to help you simplify weight loss, weight control, dietary habits, exercise activities and to gain and maintain general fitness.

Customize

This book is designed to help you customize dietary habits and exercise activities to fit you as an individual, your goals, needs, wants and lifestyle.

Gain a basic understanding

This book is designed to help you gain a basic understanding of what can be done to help you take control of your weight.

Give you ideals

This book is designed to help you get the ideals that you can apply to weight loss and weight maintenance, that will enhance your lifestyle, instead of degrading it.

Realistic goals

This book is designed to give you a realistic outlook and usable means to maintain weight goals for the rest of your life.

Understand moderation

This book is designed to help you gain an understanding of how to moderately reduce calories and increase activity, in order to lose weight without having to give up every food or activity you enjoy.

Lifestyle activities

This book is designed to help you gain knowledge of how to realistically incorporate extra activity into your lifestyle, within the time limits that you have.

Gain enjoyment

Last but not least this book is also designed to help you understand that you can incorporate activities that you enjoy doing, instead of having to force yourself to exercise at every workout.

Basically, this book will be many various things to many various people. Each person is an individual, and you will determine what this book is, for you.

WHAT THIS BOOK IS NOT

I want to make sure that you understand that I'm not claiming this is a fix-all book. So here is a list of the primary things this book is not:

Not a bodybuilding guide

This book is not a bodybuilding guide. Although bodybuilders could use the principles of weight loss in this book, it is not designed to show you the extreme muscle building exercises, that would be required for you to be a professional bodybuilder.

Not a guide for fitness models

This book is not a guide for fitness models. Again this book concentrates on general fitness, and not the development of a perfectly proportioned physique, that would be required for you to be a fitness model.

Not a guide for extreme athletes

This book is not a guide for extreme athletes such as MMA fighters, professional ballplayers or other extreme sports participants.

Not a quick fix

This book is not a quick-fix fad diet system, that promises extreme weight losses in very short periods of time.

Not a prearranged program

This book is not an extreme or prearranged exercise system. You will develop your own activities.

Not an endorsement

This book is not a sales pitch or endorsement for any product or service.

Now that we've covered a little bit about this book, I want to make sure that you understand this book is about simplifying, customizing and hopefully even getting you to enjoy the weight-loss process.

Now let's get to the meat and potatoes. **Hey!** Not those meat and potatoes. Let me rephrase that. Let's get started on the next section.

GENERAL WEIGHT LOSS ISSUES

In this section we are going to cover generalized issues that concern all aspects of weight loss including: healthy weight evaluation methods, commonalities of fit people, Possible causes of weight gain, general guidelines, weight loss do's, and weight loss don'ts.

HEALTHY WEIGHT EVALUATION METHODS

There is various methods used to evaluate healthy body weight. I just want to make sure that you understand these are *guidelines*, and what is healthy for one person may not be healthy for another. As you will see I have strong opinions for some of these methods, but I will try to give you unbiased information. Some of the methods used to evaluate healthy body weight are as follows:

Body fat percentage test

These are test or methods used to determine the overall percent of body fat you carry on your body, as opposed to other body tissue and components such as: muscle, skin, bone, organs, etc. These test can be performed utilizing tools or methods such as: skin fold calipers, pinch test, underwater weighing, bioelectric impedance, and various other methods are used. But all have one purpose, to determine the percentage of body fat. I'm not going to go into great detail to describe these methods or how they are done. The methods that you can do your self, should have instructions provided with the tools that you use. The other methods you will have to seek out professionals who offer these services and will be able to describe them to you.

So what is a healthy fat percentage? This is something else that the so-called "experts" cannot seem to agree on. Common sense tells us the reason they cannot agree, is because every individual is different and that there is not one specific number that is right for everybody. Therefore we will give you a wide range for the various classifications, that most people tend to agree with.

But first let's clarify the different classifications of fat percentage ranges.

- **Essential fat classification** is the fat which you must have for the purposes of survival, you should never fall below this range.

- **Athlete classification** athletes tend to carry much lower fat percentages than the average person.

- **Fitness classification** is for the percent of body fat that is considered fit in general fitness terms.

- **Acceptable classification** is the percent of body fat that is considered average, it may not be considered fit, but is acceptable for health concerns.

- **Obese classification** this is the percentage of body fat that you are considered to be overweight or obese. This is the percentage that you need to try to stay below.

The healthy body fat percentage range for each classification are as follows:

- **Essential fat:** Women = 10-12% Men = 2-4%

- **Athletes:** Women = 14-20% Men = 6-13%

- **Fitness:** Women = 21-24% Men = 14-17%

- **Acceptable:** Women = 25-31% Men = 18-25%

- **Obese:** Women = 32% + Men = 26% +

That is the general range of body fat percentage and some of the methods used to evaluate them. Now let's look at another method of healthy weight evaluation.

Waist measurement

This is one of the simplest ways to evaluate healthy body weight. The procedure simply involves, taking a measurement around your waist, at the navel (belly button), while sucking in your stomach. The reason you suck in your stomach, is because you're going to have a tendency to do it anyway, also it helps get the muscles of the abs out of the way, producing more accurate results.

Waist measurements can be a very good indicator for health risks, because fat that you carry around your abdominal area, is the most dangerous.

The general guideline for waist measurement is that women should strive for a waist measurement below 35 inches. Men should strive for a waist measurement of below 40 inches. For optimal health, another guideline is to aim for a waist measurement that is half or below your height.

In my opinion this is probably one of the best ways to evaluate healthy weight. Simply because, it is so easy to do, very convenient and fairly accurate.

Other measurements

You can also use measurements to measure other parts of the body in order to more closely monitor whether you are gaining muscle or losing fat. Other measurement sites can include the neck, chest, biceps, thighs (upper part of the leg), and the calves. The general guideline for monitoring progress, is that you want the parts of the body that accumulate the most fat to get smaller and you want the parts of the body that do not accumulate fat to either remain the same or get slightly larger from developing muscle mass. This is a fairly accurate healthy weight measuring and monitoring technique, especially when used in conjunction with waist measurement. It can however, become tedious and slightly more complicated and time-consuming than waist measurement alone.

The next method of weight evaluation we are going to discuss is....

Scale weight

This is simply standing on a weight scale to determine how much you weigh. This is probably one of the simplest forms of weight evaluation. It can be a beneficial way of determining changes in your weight, when combined with other methods. However it only measures overall weight and does not show the differences in fat and muscle weight.

In my opinion this type of evaluation method is not very accurate when used by itself. If you cut too many calories to quickly, weight loss can come from lost muscle tissue and not fat, the scale by itself would not show this. Also if you do strenuous resistance training, weight gain could come from gaining muscle mass which could actually lower your fat percentage making you more healthy, but again the scale would not show this, it would simply show weight gain.

Photos

This is simply taking photographs periodically, just like the before and after photos you see in magazine ads for supplements. This can be a very effective way to visually see progress over an extended period of time. However, photos may not show small amounts of progress, therefore photos should be used in conjunction with some other healthy weight measurement technique.

To take a photo you would generally dress in the least amount of clothing possible, whatever you're comfortable with and depending on who will see the photos. Photos should be taken from the front, side and back so that you get a better overall view. You want to be sure to take all photos in the same pose and with the same amount of tension within the muscles of the body. One suggestion for this is to place your hands on your hips and tense your muscles as hard as possible in every photo. Photos are generally taken every 30 days so that they can be compared and monitor progress. Utilize some other healthy weight measurement tool or technique in conjunction with photos, so that you can monitor progress more frequently.

The last weight evaluation method I would like to discuss with you is....

Body mass index (BMI)

In my opinion this is the most worthless evaluation method ever created. But, to try to give you unbiased information I will force myself to discuss it.

Body mass index or BMI for short is a calculation that takes height and weight and calculates it into an index number. For long-distance runners, people who have very little muscle mass, and others in general who do not do any type of resistance, not just an exercise but in their everyday life, this can be a very accurate healthy weight evaluation tool.

However, because the BMI does not take into consideration weight that comes from any type of muscle mass, it is virtually useless in evaluating healthy weight in individuals who have very much muscle mass. Many people non-athletes and athletes alike, who participate in resistance training, with very low body fat percentages including below 8%, are shown to be obese according to the BMI.

I know, I said I'd try to be unbiased, but anyone who does any type of resistance, that may cause muscle mass, cannot be properly evaluated with a BMI. This includes people who are simply carrying extra weight from being obese. Obese people generally have very high muscle mass in their legs and calves, from carrying the extra weight. And it enrages me at how many professionals, including doctors still use the BMI to evaluate peoples weight related health.

Now that I've got that out of my system lets take a look at....

COMMONALITIES OF FIT PEOPLE

Every single fit person has certain things in common, that they either do or don't do. So let's take a look at some of these things they share.

Body movement

Every single person that is fit moves their body in some way or another. Some move rapidly, some move slowly, some move gracefully, some move purposely, some move aggressively, etc.

Weight trainers move weights with their body, sometimes slowly, sometimes explosively. Bodybuilders move weights with their body for the purposes of building massively huge muscles. Strength trainers move weights with their bodies for the purposes of developing maximum strength. Strength endurance trainers move weights with their body for the purposes of developing strength endurance and toning their bodies.

Tai chi and Chi gong participants move their body slowly and gracefully through various forms while coordinating their breathing with the movements, for the purposes of stimulating internal organs and gaining a balanced and peaceful mind.

Yogis or yoga participants move their body through various resisted or balancing poses while also coordinating their breathing with the movements. They do this for the purposes of flexibility, mobility, and a relaxed, focused and peaceful mind.

Pilates and calisthenics participants move their bodies through various bodyweight resistance exercises. They do this for the purposes of strengthening, toning and building strength endurance.

Are you getting the point yet? There is not a specific way that you have to move your body, but you do have to move your body in some way or another in order to lose weight and gain fitness.

Now let's look at something else they have in common.

Breath control

Every fit person out there controls their breath or breathing pattern at one point or another especially during exercise. Breathing is a very important aspect of everyday life that most people take for granted.

As we mentioned earlier tai chi, Chi gong and yoga participants all coordinate their breathing with their body movements.

Even people that perform resistance training whether it's with some form of weights or bodyweight, all control their breathing in some form or another. An example is that most resistance trainers will breathe out when they exert force against the resistance.

Some cultures believe that every living being has a predetermined number of breaths, and that if you breathe more deeply and slower that you will be healthier and live longer. Some people believe that doing breathing exercises such as power breathing, can by itself improve health and help with weight loss. No matter what your belief, you should realize that breathing plays an important role in every aspect of your life including weight loss and fitness.

Dietary habits control

I'm sure every one of us knows someone who seems to be able to eat anything they want and not gain weight. But in reality, every fit person may not always watch what they eat, but they do have overall good dietary habits.

Most will eat bad foods in moderation, will eat slowly and thoroughly chew their food, will stop eating when they feel full and so on. Bottom line if you are going to lose and maintain your weight you must be in control of your eating and dietary habits.

The last and possibly the most important thing that fit people have in common is....

Enjoy what they do to get fit

What I mean by this is that most fit individuals enjoy whatever it is they do to get fit, whether it is exercise or lifestyle activity.

Bodybuilders, strength trainers and other resistance trainers do not lift weights because they hate lifting weights. If asked, most would admit to enjoying lifting weights, whether it is the process or the challenge.

Marathon runners do not run marathons because they hate to run. Most runners enjoy running, again either for the activity itself or the challenge of it. The point is most people that are either fit or good at something enjoy not only the benefits but also the process itself. This is something that you need to keep in mind and realize that if you're having to force yourself every single time you exercise, it's time to find a different activity.

See if you can't think of other things that fit people have in common, and try to incorporate them into your daily life. Now let's move on to....

POSSIBLE CAUSES OF WEIGHT GAIN

In order for you to take control of your life and lose weight, it is very important for you to have a basic understanding of where your weight gain came from. There is many possible causes for weight gain we are going to list a few of them here.

Eating too much

This is when you eat more calories than you can burn throughout the day or when you eat so much at one meal you stretch your stomach. The reasons for this could be many including but not limited to: eating too fast, not eating frequently enough, simply not being able to control eating, etc.

Being inactive

This is where you lead a sedentary lifestyle where you do very little movement or activities. Reasons for this include: lack of energy, lack of time, lack of motivation, lack of ideals or knowledge and various other reasons which we will explore in later sections.

Eating overly processed or chemical laden foods

Our bodies do not know what to do with all of these foreign chemicals. The rise of obesity can be directly linked to when companies first started putting all of the additives and chemicals in food.

Stress

Stress creates a chemical in the body that is called cortisol, which has been shown in studies to cause weight gain. So as you see, a weight loss program that is not simple and causes extra stress, could be counterproductive.

Hormone imbalances

Some people have hormonal imbalances within their bodies that causes them to gain weight. Conditions that may cause hormonal imbalances include but is not limited to: hyperthyroidism, polycystic ovary syndrome (PCOS),etc. This is why it is very important to get a medical evaluation before starting any weight loss program.

Water retention

Some people can be overweight simply because of excess water within their body. Some causes of this include but are not limited to: excess salt intake, hormonal imbalances, health conditions, etc.

Food sensitivity

There are some people that have an allergy or special sensitivity to certain foods that can cause them to gain weight when they eat this food.

Drug side effects

Some prescription and nonprescription drugs can cause weight gain. It is very important that if you are taking any medication or drugs, that you find out what the possible side effects are and consult with a medical professional.

Depression

Sometimes this can be linked with cortisol, sometimes it causes separate effects such as overeating or other weight gaining problems. If you believe you have depression you need to seek professional medical attention.

Aging

The process of aging can cause weight gain. It is estimated that after a certain age people gain 1 pound of fat a year, just around internal organs alone. However you should not allow this to cause you worry, because it has been shown that proper dietary habits and an active lifestyle can slow and even reverse age related weight gain and the aging process.

Genetics

These are the traits that you inherit from your parents, relatives and other ancestors. It has been shown, that people with overweight parents, are more likely to be overweight themselves. Which means that weight gain can be hereditary. Again you should not allow this to cause you undo concern, because like aging, genetic weight problems can be overcome with proper dietary habits and an active lifestyle.

These are some of the causes of weight gain. There is many more too numerous to list here, most others come in the form of some disease or other medical condition. Therefore it is very important for you to get a medical evaluation, when you rapidly gain weight, and before you start any weight loss program.

Now let's take a look at some....

GENERAL GUIDELINES

This is generalized information that you may find useful. Keep in mind that these are only guidelines, and you should determine how you use them. Remember every individual is unique.

METHODS USED FOR WEIGHT LOSS

There is a great number of methods you can use to lose and manage weight. Following is a list of some of the most common methods and a brief description. We will get into more detailed descriptions in upcoming sections.

Calorie reduction

This is where you reduce the amount of calories you consume, by using one or a combination of various techniques. Some of these techniques include but are not limited to: eating less at each meal, counting calories, eliminating or substituting certain foods, following specialized diets (low-carb, low-fat, fasting, etc.), drinking no-calorie liquids before meals, eating slower in order to allow the body to register when it's full, and various other methods.

Increasing activity

This is where you increase the amount of calories you burn through physical exertion. There is also lots of various ways, methods and techniques you can utilize to increase activity. Some of these are: walking, hiking, resistance training (weights, kettle bells, club bells, bodyweight, etc.), sports, physically active games, skill training, gardening and various other methods. The important thing to remember about activity, is that it can be anything that burns more calories than you are burning now.

Eating clean

This is a method where you eliminate all of the highly processed foods, and eat only natural foods that has not been processed or had chemicals added to them. People that follow this method claim they do not have to count calories or worry about how much they eat, and their body still sheds excess fat. This is a very good and healthy way to lose and maintain weight. However, as with other methods some people will find this unrealistic and very difficult to stick to for prolonged periods of time.

Pharmaceutical drugs and supplements

This is where you utilize some form of prescription drug or over-the-counter supplement to aid in weight loss. Because of past experiences, I am not an advocate of these methods they can be unpredictable and very dangerous. If you decide you want to utilize one of these I would recommend visiting a doctor and going with the prescription weight loss pill, so that at least your doctor can monitor any side effects. Again trying to be unbiased, I have met many people who has had great success with these methods. Just be careful and do your own personal research. Remember that supplement companies are in the business to make money.

Bariatric surgery

There is a number of surgical procedures available to help treat obesity. The most common types of surgery seems to be variations on two procedures. One involves placing a band around the top of the stomach opening, in order to reduce the amount or frequency of food entry into the stomach. The second procedure involves stapling or removing part of the stomach itself, in order to reduce its size, and reduced the amount of food that can be consumed. Surgery is very risky and should be the last option, and only for severely obese individuals. You will need to consult with a medical professional who performs these types of surgeries, in order to determine whether you are a candidate who may benefit from this type of procedure.

Combination methods

This is where you use a combination of two or more of the other methods to create a calorie deficit. Simply put, a deficit is when you burn more calories than you consume. Most people claim that this is the easiest way to lose weight. In theory it is, because you can do a little bit of some of the techniques, instead of having to do a lot of one of the techniques. This is probably what everyone should be aiming for especially for the maintenance phase, controlling dietary habits and leading a more active life style. However, as we mentioned before every one is different, this method will be easier for some, but for others, when they first start it may be easier to concentrate on one problem area, until they can gain control, then add methods as they're able.

That is some of the basic methods that can be used to lose and maintain your weight. But before you can decide which methods would be best for you, you must....

DETERMINE WHAT IS RESPONSIBLE FOR YOUR WEIGHT GAIN

We discussed earlier the possible Causes of weight gain. The above causes was very generalized, in this section we are going to try to narrow them down, so that you can pinpoint your most problem areas. For example: for people who eat too much, there is generally a reason they eat too much. These reasons are what we are going to explore. The more you know about what is causing your weight problem and the reasons for these causes, the easier it will be for you to customize your weight loss lifestyle most effectively.

Everyone is different, and each individual will have different reasons for being overweight. Some people may get plenty of activity but simply consume more calories than their body can burn. Others don't necessarily, consume too many calories, but lead such an inactive lifestyle, that their bodies can not utilize all of the calories.

It is very important for you to narrow down the causes and reasons for your weight problems. If you drastically cut calories too low, your body will think it is starving, and slow its metabolism and store extra fat, making it harder to lose weight and maintain for extended periods of time. If you drastically increase activity too much or too fast, it can cause over-training, which can lead to injury or sickness and can also be very hard to maintain for extended periods of time.

Also knowing the causes and reasons that are most responsible for your weight problems, and that may be the most difficult to control, will allow you to focus primarily on correcting these problems one at a time. By focusing primarily on these main problems can make it much simpler, than trying to drastically change a whole lot of aspects of your lifestyle all at once.

Please note: that this is not a complete list of reasons for these possible causes, it would require much more space than this book provides in order to list every single possible reason. Also some reasons will be very unique to each individual. Therefore, keep in mind, the purpose of these lists, are to simply give you some ideal of possible reasons, and to open up your imagination so that you can figure out your own unique causes and reasons for your weight problem. Now let's take a look at some of these causes and the possible reasons of these causes.

Reasons for eating too much

If eating to much is one of the causes for your weight problems, then what you need to try to determine is *why* you're eating too much. Some of the reasons people eat too much are as follows:

Eating too fast: This can cause you to eat too much before your mind has time to register that it is full. Eating too fast can also stretch your stomach causing you to eat more at following meals. The habit of eating too fast can be developed through various lifestyle issues such as: Short lunch periods, busy lifestyle, being a member of a large family, military conditioning, etc.

Not chewing thoroughly: This can also be linked with eating too fast. When you do not properly chew your food it can cause problems with digestion, nutrient absorption and can also cause a delay in recognizing that you are full.

Consuming too many liquid calories: It is very easy to consume excess calories when you are drinking high calorie liquids such as: pop, sweetened juices and other sweetened or artificial drinks.

Eating too infrequently: When you go extended periods of time without eating it causes your metabolism to slow, which in return will slow the amount of calories you burn throughout the day. Not eating for extended periods of time, can also cause excessive hunger, which may cause you to eat more at later meals.

Eating too often: This is just the opposite from the above. Some people have heard that eating more often can increase metabolism and help them lose weight. However, if you consume excessive calories at each meal it will be counterproductive.

Trigger foods: Trigger foods, are foods that causes you to consume excess amounts of calories seemingly uncontrollably, for various known or unknown reasons. Trigger foods are unique to each individual. If there is a certain food that you seem to over-eat on every time you eat it, it is more than likely one of your trigger foods. Trigger foods will either have to be avoided completely, eaten very infrequently or you will have to control the portion size in some way or another.

Stress: Stress can have various different effects on people, these effects can be, excess hunger or simply eating for comfort. Stress can cause excess weight directly by causing the elevation of the hormone cortisol, or it can indirectly cause weight gain by making you eat more for one reason or another. If you believe that stress is the main problem or a partial problem of your weight problems, it is very important that you manage, eliminate or learn to deal with the stress in your life.

Social and peer pressure: There is a lot of people who'd never have a problem with eating too much, until they go out with friends or go to certain events. Whether this is from feeling they must eat as much or the same types of foods as their friends in order to fit in or because of a lack of healthy food choices at certain events or locations. If this happens very infrequently this is not much of a concern, however if a big part of your life involves these friends and social events, this can be a major problem.

Being bored: There are certain individuals who will eat out of sheer boredom. When you are bored and wanting something to do, this can create a feeling that is very similar to food cravings, this can lead to people mistaking boredom for hunger, causing them to overeat.

Loneliness: Feelings are produced through chemical changes within the brain. Events, interactions and even food can cause an elevation of these chemical responses. Some people can get a similar type of feeling from eating a certain food, as they would from talking to a loved one or friend. Therefore, certain people who lack a social life, will seek out comfort and try to re-create these feelings through food, causing them to over eat.

those are some of the reasons for overeating, if overeating is one of your primary problems, try to figure out if one of these is the reason for it. If overeating is not the problem, let's take a look at the next cause for weight gain.

Reasons for being inactive

If you lead a sedentary or inactive lifestyle this could be the primary or partial cause for your weight problems. To give you a more thorough understanding and ability to distinguish your primary problems let's take a look at some of the reasons for being inactive.

Lack of energy: Not having enough energy is the reason a lot of people give for not being more active. Lack of energy can come from: poor dietary habits, health problems, lack of interest, lack of motivation and even lack of activity. That last one confuses a lot of people, but it's an actual fact, that some people don't necessarily lack the energy, but instead have a hard time getting started. Sometimes if you will slowly start a easy simple exercise such as walking, your energy level will actually increase.

Injury or medical conditions: It is easy for people to say in order to lose weight you must simply perform exercises such as walking or running. However if you have a medical condition or injury that prevents you from doing certain exercises, then it is easier said than done. You need to be sure that you do not worsen the injury or condition and clear any activity with a medical professional. But you should keep in mind, that losing weight does not require you to do a specific exercise or workout. You can sometimes work around the injury or medical condition. To increase activity you simply, need to move the body parts you are capable of moving, more often.

Lack of interest: Some people hear about the exercises and workouts they must perform in order to become fitter, and they are just not interested in any of them. As I've mentioned earlier activity for weight loss does not have to be any specific form or type. You must find an activity that interests you and that you enjoy doing. If you are currently inactive, then any activity will be beneficial. Remember even the simple act of walking outside to look at birds, will burn more calories than sitting in a chair and looking at birds through the window.

Lack of a social life: Some people are inactive because they do not like doing things alone, and they have very little friends to do things with. It is very unlikely that someone will come knocking on your door begging to be your friend. Get out, and go to the park, mall or some other location, walk around and start a conversation with people whenever possible. This will kill two birds with one stone, so to speak, not only will you become more active through walking around, but also you may make new friends through the conversations you start. For those of you who are chronically shy, you may have to start slowly, such as a simple hello, and build to longer conversations. I know you can do it, because I have faith in you.

Lack of time: It is very easy for the self proclaimed "gurus" to constantly tell people that everyone has the same amount of time in the day. In reality, everyone is a unique individual who has unique duties and responsibilities that take up different amounts of time for each person. But remember, we are not talking about specific exercises or workouts, we are talking about activity which can come from anywhere including daily lifestyles and work. Another topic I want to bring up at this point, is that most “experts” and “gurus” tell you, that you must exercise for a specific amount of time, what they don’t tell you is that that time does not have to be continuous or all at once. It has been proven through various studies that a number of shorter activities are just as beneficial or even possibly more beneficial than longer continuous workouts.

Depression: Depression can cause people to lose interest in activities that they once enjoyed. People with depression find it hard to even function through daily life, much less having to cope with weight loss issues. Depression can come from another source and cause you to become overweight, or being overweight itself can lead to depression. Depression is a very serious condition, that must be taken seriously. If you cannot figure out the cause and overcome depression by yourself, you must seek professional medical attention.

That is some of the reasons for being inactive now let’s take a look at another cause of weight gain.

Reasons for stress

Stress is a very major factor of weight gain that many people fail to consider when they're trying to lose weight. The primary product of stress that causes weight gain is the hormone called cortisol. However, being stressed by itself can cause other factors of weight gain such as overeating, lack of energy, filling the lack of ability to deal with extra activity, and various other factors. So let's take a look at a list of some of the reasons of stress.

Work: Work related stress can come in many forms including: An overbearing boss, feeling like you're doing most of the work to make somebody else a living, not getting along with coworkers, not being paid adequately for the work you do, or simply hating the job you do.

Financial concerns: Financial related stress can include: Being unable to adequately support your family, becoming in debt, not being able to take vacations, not being able to purchase certain items, worrying about whether or not you're going to be able to pay all of your Bills, etc.

Relationship concerns: Relationship related stress can come in many forms including: Not feeling adequate or good enough for your partner, beliefs that your partner may be cheating, partners added financial responsibilities, perceived or actual expectancies of your partner and various other factors.

Family and social concerns: Feeling like an outsider, peer pressure, feeling like you must do certain things to be liked or accepted, feeling like you are the one responsible for all entertainment ideals and activities, feeling like you cannot be yourself and various other factors.

Medical reasons: Like the others these comes in various forms such as: Worrying about a medical condition, feeling that your doctor is over medicating you and giving you a medication that you don't feel you need, feeling like your doctor does not listen to you, financial concerns for medical bills, lack of medical insurance, worrying about a family member's illness, and so on.

Fitness concerns: This includes stress factors such as: Poor self-esteem, confidence, social status, health issues, unrealistic diets, unrealistic exercise programs, not knowing what to do, knowing what to do but not knowing how to do it, conflicting information and many more.

Remember that stress can come from many various places, forms and factors. It is very important that you learn to eliminate, manage or deal with stress within your daily life. It is also very important that you do not cause extra undue stress, by trying to stick with an unrealistic and complicated weight loss program.

Reasons for hormone imbalances

Certain hormones are very important for weight loss and weight management. Human growth hormone (HGH) is a hormone that is produced naturally in the body and when something causes it to be lowered, it can cause weight gain and muscle loss. Cortisol is a hormone we discussed earlier that can be elevated by stress and can cause weight gain. Insulin is a hormone that helps control blood sugar, an imbalance of this can cause weight gain as well as numerous other problems. That is just the few examples of certain hormones. We are not going to list every hormone and every possible imbalance it would be too extensive for this book. But we will list some of the causes of general hormone imbalances.

Improper nutrition: Certain chemicals in foods or a deficiency in certain nutrients can cause hormone imbalances.

Medical conditions: Certain medical conditions such as diabetes, hyperthyroidism and numerous other medical conditions can cause hormone imbalances.

Excessive alcohol use: Excessive alcohol use can cause liver damage and numerous other illnesses and medical conditions including hormone imbalances.

Tobacco use: Tobacco contains many chemicals and toxins too numerous to list here, any number of which can cause hormone imbalances as well as other diseases and illnesses.

Drug use: Every drug, prescription, nonprescription, legal or illegal, have some side effects. Some of these side effects can include hormone imbalances.

Over-training: When you do strenuous exercise without allowing an adequate amount of time to recover, your muscles continue to break down without being able to repair themselves. This can cause many problems including injuries, illnesses and you guessed it, hormone imbalances.

The only way to truly know whether you have any hormone imbalances is to have medical test run by a medical professional. Therefore, if you feel you may have a hormone imbalance that is causing your weight problem consult your physician. Now let's move on to the next issue.

Reasons for water retention

Water retention can make you appear to be overweight, can make you feel puffy, bloated and flat-out miserable. So let's take a look at some of the reasons that may cause water retention.

Excessive salt intake: The primary culprit in salt that causes water retention is sodium. This is actually a needed nutrient but in excess it can cause various medical conditions including high blood pressure, heart problems and water retention. Athletes are sometimes given salt tablets on very hot days in order to help them retain water to prevent dehydration and heat stroke.

Medical issues: Certain medical conditions can also cause you to retain water, heart problems and kidney problems can both cause you to retain water. So it's very important that if you have a lot of water retention, you check with your doctor to make sure it is not caused by a serious problem.

Improper nutrition: Improper nutrition can also make you retain water. This is not just from excessive sodium but can also be caused from nutrient deficiencies or excessive amounts of other nutrients.

Women's monthly cycle: I am not a doctor, and being a man I am not even going to pretend I am knowledgeable in this area. I do know that many women experience bloating and water retention during monthly cycles, I also know that this is a normal part of a woman's life.

That is some of the reasons for water retention. Moving right along now to reasons for food sensitivity.

Reasons for food sensitivity

Food sensitivity have many different forms, reactions and causes, here is a small list.

Allergies: Certain people are allergic to certain types of food some known and some unknown. Some reactions can be very dangerous, some reactions can be mild and sometimes reactions can either directly or indirectly cause weight gain.

Intolerance: Some people have a certain reaction to foods that is not called an allergy but rather intolerance. The most common is lactose intolerant, where people cannot drink milk or other dairy products. There are other intolerances that may not be so common. For example, some people that consume a large amount of artificial sweetener, will tend to have greater cravings and eat more at later times in the day which can lead to weight gain. If you have switched to diet pop or some other artificially sweetened product and seemed to be eating more and still not losing weight, you may have an intolerance to the artificial sweetener.

Drastic change in food types: This can come in the form of either a geographical move or a drastic dietary change. Some people in the military experience this, when consuming MRE's (meals ready to eat) or have to eat food from a different culture or country. Drastic change in foods can lead to various problems affecting digestion and metabolism both of which can lead to weight gain.

Drug side effects

The reasons for drug side effects are too numerous and out of my qualification range. There for in this section instead of listing reasons we will list some of the possible side effects that may affect weight.

Excessive hunger: Some side effects of certain drugs may be excess hunger, which causes you uncontrollable cravings and makes you eat more than you normally would. This can definitely cause weight gain.

Slowed metabolism: Another side effect of drugs can cause your metabolism to slow down, which in return will cause you to burn less calories throughout the time you are taking that drug. This again can cause weight gain even though you may not be consuming any more calories than normal.

Hormone imbalances: As we mentioned earlier when we were discussing hormone imbalances, this can be a possible side effect of drugs.

Water retention: We've also mentioned this earlier. Certain drugs can cause you to retain more water than normal.

Source of stress: Certain drugs can cause extra stress either as a side effect, or from different worries or stress about drugs that we talked about earlier.

Depression: Certain drugs may cause depression again either directly from a side effect, or simply from drug-related issues such as becoming depressed about the amount of drugs you have to take in order to lead a normal life.

Since were ending with depression, let's let that lead us into the reasons for depression.

Reasons for depression

There is many reasons for depression I cannot possibly list them all and I'm not even going to claim that I know even half of them much less all of them. So I will just give a partial list here to give you an idea.

Low self-esteem: Low self-esteem and lack of confidence can start out mild, but when it goes on for prolonged periods of time without being overcome it can lead to depression.

Lack of a social life: This may or may not stem from low self-esteem. It has been said that "no man is an island unto himself" which in simple terms means everyone needs someone. Without someone in your life to talk to, depend on and simply communicate openly with, can quickly lead to depression.

Lack of control in your life: Whether this is perceived or actual, it can be very devastating. When someone feels that they have no control over what goes on in their life they can very quickly become depressed.

Family and social pressure: This can come in the form of family members having unrealistic expectations or the person themselves feels responsible for certain aspects of the entire family. Either way, when they can not live up to or meet these expectations or responsibilities it can cause depression.

Loss: Whether this is the loss of a person, pet, or even an item it can be very devastating. Everyone will handle and even perceive loss differently. Some people just cannot handle certain types of loss and quickly fall into depression.

Financial concerns: Money means different things to different people primarily depending on whether you have money or not. Some people who are struggling to make ends meet, can feel overcome by financial burdens, and may even start to feel inadequate in different aspects of their life which again can quickly lead to depression.

As I mentioned earlier this is only a partial list, and I have no medical degree so I am not going to go into much depth about this subject. The only thing I can stress is that if you feel you have depression consult a medical professional. Now let's talk a little bit about aging.

Aging

The reasons for aging is not exactly a mystery, it's simply because we get older. Therefore similar to what we did with drug side effects, instead of listing reasons we are going to list some of the weight related problems that the aging process causes.

Slowed metabolism: As we age our metabolism slows and we burn less and less calories. Some of this slowdown occurs directly because of the aging process itself, other causes of this slowdown is indirectly linked to other factors caused by aging.

Hormone changes: Certain hormones including but not limited to HGH and testosterone slowly decrease as we age. As we discussed earlier a decrease in these hormones can cause weight gain and muscle loss.

Age-related ailments: As we age we develop or at least increase the chances of developing age-related ailments such as: arthritis, bursitis, vision loss, hearing loss, heart problems, and numerous other elements. This can lead to a less active lifestyle and weight gain.

Internal fat increase: As I mentioned earlier, after a certain age people start to develop fat around and in their internal organs, this is usually on average around a pound a year.

Muscle atrophy: As we age we lose muscle either directly because of the aging process or indirectly because of the drop in physical activity.

Irregularities in digestion: As we age our bodies find it harder to process the foods we eat, which can lead to irregularities within our digestive systems.

As I mentioned before age-related problems can be slowed and in some cases even reversed to a certain degree through developing better dietary and active lifestyle habits. Now let's move on to the last cause of weight gain.

Genetics

Like other issues we have discussed, the reasons for genetics is obvious, it comes from your genes. Therefore instead of listing reasons I will give you a list of possible signs that your weight problems may be genetic.

Overweight relatives: If other members of your family are overweight especially your parents, weight problems may be genetic and run in your family. Be absolutely sure, that you're not just using this as an excuse, if overweight members of your family also have poor dietary habits and lead sedentary lifestyles, then the weight problem may be from these issues and not genetics.

Lack of progress from traditional weight-loss programs: If you have followed realistic programs that has been proven to work for others, religiously, but failed to get adequate results, this might possibly be a sign that some of your weight problems stem from genetics.

You have been overweight your entire life: If you have had weight problems your entire life, despite proper nutrition and activities, this may be a sign that your weight problems are hereditary.

Even if your weight problems do stem from genetics, all hope is not lost. Even though it may be more difficult, and you might not be able to get the same results such as professional athletes you can still attain a healthy weight and other benefits from following a healthier and more active lifestyle.

Now let's move on and list some....

WEIGHT-LOSS DO'S

Let's discuss some of the things that you can do to improve your weight loss success. The following list is things that you should do or incorporate into your weight-loss lifestyle or program whenever possible.

Do get a checkup

You should check with your doctor, before starting any weight loss program. It is very important to make sure that your current weight problems are not caused by any medical condition. It is also important to make sure that any dietary or activity changes, will not create or worsen any medical problems.

Do Simplify

You should simplify the weight-loss process as much as possible. The Simpler you make it, the easier it will be to follow, stick to and maintain. By keeping it simple, you can also avoid adding any undue stress, that could be counterproductive.

Do customize

The most effective weight loss program will be the one that fits you. You should customize your weight loss program to fit your own wants, needs, abilities, willingness, likes, dislikes, etc.

Do maintain consistency

For any dietary or activity change to work, you must actually do them. Simplify and customize a program, that your willing to do. Try to incorporate daily habits, no matter how small. Remember even 10 to 15 minutes a day for three to five days a week, is going to be much better and get more efficient results, then an hour or longer program that you're only capable of forcing yourself to do once a month, would ever get.

Do create a lifestyle

Remember you're not just wanting to lose the weight, but also *maintain* this weight loss. Any changes you make needs to fit your lifestyle. You want to become a fitter healthier *you*, you do not want to become a completely different person who you do not recognize or like.

Do make it enjoyable

The more enjoyable an activity is, the more likely you are to do it. The more enjoyable a food product is, the more likely you are to eat it. When something is enjoyable to you, you find ways to incorporate it into your lifestyle, instead of making excuses for why you can't.

Do make moderate adjustments

Make gradual changes within your lifestyle that is easy for you to incorporate, stick to and maintain. This is not a race, make changes at your own pace that you are comfortable with. Even if it takes you an entire year to lose the weight, you will be more likely to be able to maintain that weight. If you try to make drastic changes, to quickly, that you cannot maintain you may be able to lose weight rapidly, but you will not be able to maintain this for extended periods of time, and one year from now, you would be worse off than you are now.

Do work on biggest problem areas first

If you narrow down to your most problem area whether it's a dietary or activity problem, you can concentrate on this problem alone, making it much simpler to achieve. Also when you correct your biggest problem you will gain confidence, and know that you are capable of achieving weight loss, making the rest of the changes much simpler.

Do be flexible

No dietary or exercise program is written in stone. Life is very unpredictable, there will be unforeseen circumstances that will arise. Remember, you are in charge, make sure you are flexible enough, to work around these circumstances or any other obstacles you may encounter.

Do allow yourself to adapt

You always hear the so-called "experts" talking about adaptation like it is a bad thing. They're always telling you to constantly change your program so that your body will not adapt. Your body will adapt to dietary and activity changes, but that is a good thing. Adapting is how your body becomes better and more efficient. You may need to slightly modify or change your program every now and then, but it does not have to be drastic and constant changes. You can change your program when you become bored with it or it stops producing the results you desire, but you are ultimately in charge, so change it when you want to. When someone tells you "your body is going to adapt if you keep doing that", look them in the eye and say "good, that's why I'm doing it".

Do be patient

Remember, this is not a race. By making gradual changes, you will achieve gradual results, but they are more likely to be permanent. Drastic weight-loss will be very hard to keep off. Every individual will be unique, just remember to keep it simple and customized. You may have fluctuations in your weight loss results, but a general guideline, is to lose 1-2 pounds or less a week, but no more than this. Anything over 1-2 pounds a week, will be very difficult to maintain for extended periods of time.

Do use accurate weight evaluation methods

Use healthy weight evaluation methods, that are accurate and fit your lifestyle. Body fat percentage test and waist measurement is in my opinion the most effective. The scale is adequate, but may not be an accurate method when used by itself, especially if you incorporate any type of resistance training.

There are some weight loss do's to get you started. But remember this is your program, so you may want to incorporate some of your own do's.

WEIGHT LOSS DON'TS

Now lets take a look at some of the things you should not do, to increase your weight loss success. The following list is some things that you should avoid or not incorporate into your weight-loss lifestyle or program. Most of these are simply the opposites of the do's, we'll look at them as don'ts, in order to give you a different perspective.

Don't over complicate

Weight-loss is not rocket science. It may not always be extremely easy, but you should simplify it as much as you can. The more complicated you make your program or lifestyle changes, the easier it will be for you to avoid doing or make excuses why you can't.

Don't use a program designed for someone else

What works for one person, may not work for another. Do not incorporate or follow lifestyle changes or a program that is unrealistic or does not fit your goals or lifestyle. If you want to be lean, with very little muscle mass, you should not follow a body builders program. If you want to be very muscular, you should not follow a marathon runners program. And if you want to be somewhere in between for general fitness and health, your program will have to be balanced accordingly. Remember customize all changes and programs to fit you.

Don't be non-consistent

Sporadic, hit and miss programs will not give you efficient, consistent results. Being consistent with your dietary and activity changes, even in moderation will give you much more efficient and beneficial results.

Don't use a program that does not fit you

If you have to change every aspect of your lifestyle and who you are, in order to follow a program, that is the wrong program for you. You should not have to change who you are in order to lose weight. If you are an intense person high intensity exercise may be for you. If you are laid-back and easy-going, you may want to stick with less intense programs. There is multiple ways to do everything.

Don't think of weight loss as punishment

In high school, when you did something wrong, coaches would make you run or do push-ups for punishment. As a child when you acted up, your parents may not have allowed you to eat a food that you liked, to punish you for acting up. You're not in high school anymore and you're no longer a child. When you view dietary and activity changes as punishment, they become very difficult to do, especially when you don't feel you've done anything you should be punished for. Activity that you incorporate into your lifestyle should be fun. Foods that you allow yourself to eat should not just be nutritious, but also taste good, and be enjoyable to eat.

Don't take on more than you can handle

The only person that knows what you are truly capable of doing and what you're willing to do, is you. Making drastic unrealistic changes will only set you up for failure. Incorporate changes moderately at your own pace so that you're capable of adjusting to them and maintaining them for the rest of your life.

Don't be rigid

Being too rigid and inflexible with your dietary and activity changes, will not allow you to overcome life's emergencies or unforeseen circumstances. If you have designed a 30 minute program, and one day, find yourself with only 15 minutes, don't be afraid to shorten your workout for that day, instead of just missing it entirely. If you find yourself someplace that only has high calorie food choices, try to adjust the amount and portions, to compensate. Remember everything fits in moderation, the only time it truly becomes bad for us is when we become excessive and consume or do too much or to little.

Don't be afraid of adaptation

Adaptation is the way your body overcomes its limitations. Without adaptation we would never be able to get stronger, healthier, faster or lose weight. Don't just change your program simply because you're afraid your body is going to adapt. You want it to adapt. Once your body adapts to weight loss, it becomes easier to maintain.

Don't be afraid to change

This one kind of goes hand-in-hand with the one above. In the same aspect that you shouldn't be afraid of adaptation, you also should not be afraid to change your program when you need to or want to. Doing the same thing over and over, can become very boring. Remember, there is multiple ways to do everything, so you have multiple choices to choose from. If you become bored, or your body adapts but you want more or different results, feel free to change or modify your program in any way you need to or want to.

Don't be impatient

This reminds me of a couple of old sayings, "good things come to those who wait" and "Patience is a virtue" these happen to be two of my favorites. It is unlikely that you are going to see instant results. Remember we are not trying to go for the quick-fix programs that do not last. We want results we can realistically maintain for the rest of our lives. When you incorporate changes gradually and moderately each change may not make a huge difference, but when you keep adding changes, and continue to maintain these changes, they will have a cumulative effect. If you have patience and persistence, I believe you will be very surprised at the results you can achieve and maintain.

Don't use unreliable weight evaluation methods

As we discussed earlier, there are some bodyweight evaluation methods that are just simply unreliable or inefficient. The weight scale has its place, and can be beneficial, however it may not be accurate when used by itself, especially if you're doing any type of training that produces muscle mass. You know by now how I feel about the body mass index (BMI), but I will say it again. In my opinion the BMI is the most worthless weight evaluation tool ever created. It does not take into consideration the differences in weight that comes from different sources such as skin, muscle, bone, water, organs, etc. Therefore, for anybody other than someone who is very skinny, it is not an accurate assessment of healthy weight. I will say this again also, everyone is different. A healthy weight for one person may not be a healthy weight for another person. A weight that is too heavy for one person may be another persons ideal weight.

That wraps up this section, in the following sections we're going to get into the actual techniques and principles that you may be able to incorporate and apply in order to lose weight.

DIETARY CONCERNS

In this section I am going to tell you to stop eating all the food you enjoy and count every calorie that enters your mouth. Just kidding! Actually in this section I am going to try to give you realistic ways to modify your dietary habits to lose weight. So if dietary concerns is your biggest reason for being overweight this section may be where you want to start.

Remember you want to customize and simplify. Use as many or as few of these tips and techniques as you need or want. You can either choose what you feel will be your hardest problem to correct, and work on it by itself, until you have corrected it or you can start with easier problems to correct. The choice is yours, this is your program that you will customize to fit your needs. So customize and simplify and make it work for you.

GENERAL NUTRITION INFORMATION

I'm going to give you some generalized nutritional information here primarily concerning the macronutrients: protein, carbohydrates and fat's. I'm going to avoid going into too much detail and will also try to avoid unnecessary scientific and medical jargon. This is just some information nuggets, that you may find useful and be able to utilize to your benefit.

Macronutrient calorie comparisons

This is how many calories each macronutrient contains per gram. I've also listed the calories per gram that is contained in alcohol for informational purposes.

- **Protein:** 1 gram = 4 calories
- **Carbohydrates:** 1 gram = 4 calories
- **Fat:** 1 gram = 9 calories
- **Alcohol:** 1 gram = 7 calories

As you can see fat and alcohol has more calories per gram than protein or carbohydrates. Therefore products containing these should be consumed in moderation.

Macronutrient purposes

Each macronutrient serve specific functions and purposes. Here is a list of some of these purposes and functions.

Protein: Proteins are made up of amino acids, which are the building blocks of the human body. Protein is essential for the growth, repair, maintenance and replacement of body tissue such as: skin, muscle, organs, hair, nails, etc. Protein is also essential to the structure of red blood cells, proper functioning of antibodies that resist infection and for regulating enzymes and hormones.

Carbohydrates: The primary purpose of carbohydrates is to provide your body with energy for activities that last less than 20 minutes. There are two primary types of carbohydrates.

- Simple carbohydrates: Also known as simple sugars. These types of carbohydrates basically burn off very quickly and are responsible for immediate short-term energy.

- Complex carbohydrates: These are the carbohydrates that burn more slowly and are responsible for the longer sustained energy lasting up to 20 minutes.

Fat: The primary function of fat is to provide energy after the body has burned off the energy from carbohydrates, generally with activities lasting longer than 20 minutes. Fat also help maintain the body's temperature, protect body tissues and organs and also carry the fat soluble vitamins: A, D, E and K throughout the body that it collects from food sources. There are four primary types of fats.

- Polyunsaturated fat: This is a good fat that tends to lower overall blood cholesterol.

- Monounsaturated fat: This is another good fat that tends to lower LDL cholesterol levels (LDL cholesterol is considered the bad cholesterol).

- Saturated fat: This is a less healthy fat and tends to increase blood cholesterol levels. This fat should be reduced and should not make up more than 10% of your overall daily calories.

- Trans fat: Also known as trans-fatty acids. This is a man-made fat that is extremely unhealthy. It has been linked to various health-related ailments and conditions. Some states are in the process of or already have banned food products that contain trans fats. Trans fat should be completely eliminated and avoided whenever possible.

Macronutrient sources

Here is a list of food sources where these macronutrients can be found. This is only a generalized and partial list, I cannot possibly list every single food available. It is just to give you a generalized ideal of some of the food sources, so that you can make better choices.

Protein sources: Meat, fish, milk, and eggs are complete proteins that have all of the essential amino acids. Other sources of proteins are whole grains, beans, rice, corn, legumes, peas, oatmeal and peanut butter.

Carbohydrate sources: Simple carbohydrates (simple sugars) are found in fruits, milk and sweetened food products.

Complex carbohydrates can be found in whole grains, flour, bread, rice, oats, corn, legumes and potatoes.

Fat sources: Polyunsaturated fat can be found in fish, flax seeds, flax oil, walnuts, safflower, corn, sunflower, soy, cottonseed, and other vegetable oils.

Monounsaturated fat: Can be found in olive oil, peanut oil, canola oils, avocados and most nuts.

Saturated fat: can be found in red meat, poultry, butter, whole milk, tropical oils and fried foods.

Trans fat: This fat is most commonly found in commercially prepared foods such as: crackers, cookies, cakes, doughnuts, french-fries, shortenings and some margarines.

DIETARY METHODS USED TO LOSE WEIGHT

Here I will describe some of the methods used to lose weight, some traditional and some not so traditional. These are simply guidelines for these methods, you can use one, you can mix and match and combine elements from all of them, or you can simply find your own unique way. You may choose to use dietary methods alone or slightly modified diet habits and combine elements for activity and mental exercise, or any combination thereof. There are multiple ways to do everything, the choice is yours.

Counting calories

If you're the type of person that likes to write things down, keep track of and count things, this may be the perfect method for you. If you're the type of person that hates to write things down, keep track of and count things, then you should probably avoid this method.

Caution!: I want to give you a word of caution, if you choose to use this method. There is a minimum amount of calories that every one needs just to function and survive, this of course is going to be unique to every individual. However as a guideline, women should never drop calories below 1200 calories per day and men should never drop calories below 1800 calories per day. Remember these are only guidelines, and for most people even these could be very severe restrictions.

There is 3500 calories in a pound of stored fat. So in theory if you was to create a deficit of 3500 calories per week, you would lose 1 pound of body weight per week. Keep in mind this deficit can come from many sources including: diet, exercise or activity or any combination thereof. In order to create a 3500 calorie deficit per week, you would have to create a 500 calorie deficit per day. If you created a 1000 calorie deficit per day you could lose 2 pounds per week. You should never try to create a deficit larger than 500 - 1000 calories per day. The larger the deficit you create the harder it is going to be to maintain. This is not a race! Think about it! Even if you lost 1 pound every two weeks, wouldn't that be better than gaining weight?

There are many test available that supposedly will tell you your daily calorie requirements, these test are available through many sources including: books, magazines, online, etc. The problem with these test is that they are not 100% accurate and cannot possibly factor in every single thing you do in your daily life.

A more realistic way, is to determine whether you are gaining or maintaining your current weight. Then determine how many calories you're consuming presently, without changing anything, and then slightly and moderately, start creating a deficit based on your current calorie consumption and specific weight problem.

Low-carb dieting

Severe carbohydrate restriction is not a realistic long-term method. However, the reason I have listed it, is because moderate carb control can be very beneficial to many individuals.

Caution!: You should never try to completely eliminate all carbohydrates from your diet. Carbohydrates are necessary for survival and healthy functioning of the body. Also a high protein, high fat diet for extended periods of time can cause undue stress on internal body organs and become very unhealthy.

A lot of people get very excited when they believe they can eat all the fat and protein that they want, and still lose weight. The problem occurs when they realize that they cannot eat certain food items such as; breads, cakes, pastas, most junk food, and even certain vegetables. Again, any time you severely restrict your choices, it becomes very difficult to maintain.

A realistic way to utilize this method, would be to slightly reduce the amount of carbs you consume, primarily from man-made sources such as: white breads, junk food, high sugar juices, etc. I do not recommend eliminating vegetables, for the simple reason most people do not have a problem with eating too many vegetables. You can however make slight substitutions such as, switching to sweet potatoes instead of white potatoes.

Low-fat diets

Many individuals could benefit from eating less fat. Moderation is the key. If you are currently consuming high fat foods, and feel this may be the reason you are overweight you might want to consider this method of weight loss.

Caution!: Never try to eliminate fat completely out of your diet. As we discussed earlier there is some bad fats you can eliminate, but there is also healthy fats that is essential for the functioning of a healthy body.

A realistic approach to this method, would be to slightly start to reduce the amount of fat that you consume and replace unhealthy fats with healthier fats. Some examples: Instead of eating junk food you could snack on nuts. Replace unhealthy salad dressings with healthier oils. You could also start to eat fish or chicken two to three times per week in place of red meat.

If you choose this method just remember, to evaluate your own diet and slowly start to adjust your food choices to reduce the amount of fat you consume and eliminate unhealthy fats.

Fasting diets

This can be very dangerous and I actually would not recommend it.

However the reason I mentioned it, is because there are certain individuals who because of religion or certain beliefs, fast at certain times. Therefore I decided to discuss it.

Caution!: Fasting too frequently or for extended periods of time can lead to starvation and malnutrition. It can cause muscle wasting, tooth decay, brittle nails, hair loss and other health-related problems. Therefore you should use caution and consult a medical professional before starting any fasting program.

If your religion or other beliefs require you to fast, then you may be able to utilize this to jumpstart your weight loss lifestyle. Utilize your fast to cleanse your body and flush commercial chemicals, and when you end the fast try to start back eating a more healthy and balanced diet. Try to avoid as much of the chemical laden foods as possible.

Vegetarian diet

This is another method that may be viable because of a religion or certain beliefs. If you can do without meat and other animal products this may be a very beneficial method for you.

Caution!: The primary concern with vegetarianism is the lack of protein. As we mentioned earlier protein is a very important part of a healthy, functional body. It is very important for vegetarians to consume non-animal sources of protein such as whole grains, rice, corn, nuts, and other sources that we mentioned before.

If you are not currently a vegetarian, the most realistic way for you to become a vegetarian, would be too slowly and moderately cut down on the meats and other animal products that you eat. It is unrealistic for you to go from, one day eating high amounts of meats and dairy products, to the next day not eating any. Remember, moderately change and modify your dietary lifestyle, until you reach your goal.

Semi-vegetarian

This may be a more realistic approach for individuals who do not want to completely eliminate meat and dairy products. A semi-vegetarian only eliminates red meat. Therefore semi-vegetarians receive some of the same health benefits as vegetarians but still retain a higher source of protein. Just as above it is still very important that you eliminate red meat at your own pace and at a comfortable level, that is realistic for you to maintain.

Natural or clean eating

A lot of people mistake this for vegetarianism, however this is not true.

Natural or clean eating does not involve giving up any animal products. Instead it focuses on eliminating highly processed and chemical laden foods. It involves eating natural, organic foods that has not been sprayed, injected or modified with any chemicals, including grass fed beef and other animals.

This can be very healthy and beneficial way of eating if you can do without junk food and other highly processed foods. Another obstacle for this method is the availability and price of organic food products. In certain areas it can be very difficult to obtain organic foods without having them shipped to you. Also organic foods for some reason tend to be higher priced than other food products. The reason for this in some cases is that food manufacturers will sometimes add what is called fillers into highly processed foods lowering the price as well as nutritional value.

There are a lot of people that report a natural weight loss, reduced cravings, more energy and an overall feeling of well-being, without worrying about how much they eat, after following this eating method for a certain amount of time. As with all other methods, if you feel this method may be the best for you, it may be more realistic and easier to make changes in moderation.

Multiple meals

This method is sometimes the most easiest for people to follow. It simply involves eating more often in order to eliminate hunger. Keep in mind that you must reduce the amount of each meal, otherwise it would be counterproductive. By reducing the amount of each meal and eating more frequently, you may get many benefits including: elimination of snacking or snack foods, elevation of metabolism, better digestion and the elimination of cravings and hunger pangs. If you're the type of person who is not necessarily eating bad foods but just eating too much because of excessive hunger, this may be a viable method for you.

Combination methods

Keep in mind that there is multiple ways of doing things and that there is no single one way to do anything. Combination methods may include taking elements from different methods to create your own unique method or lifestyle. Some examples: instead of following a full-blown low-carb diet, you could eat regularly throughout the day, and stop eating carbs four to five hours before bedtime. (Eating carbs right at bedtime tends to promote them being stored as fat).

You can also eat like a vegetarian only for a certain number of days per week, this would still allow you to have red meat on certain days, but would allow you to cut down and not have it every day. (everything fits in moderation, the only time we have a problem is when we become excessive).

Another combination method you could use is to eat clean for five to six days a week, and then allow yourself either a free day or free meal once or twice a week. (A free day or meal is when you do not worry about what you eat, you can have anything you want).

The key to any of these or any other methods you choose to use is that you must modify, customize and simplify to fit you and your lifestyle and to make it the easiest and most beneficial for you. You should also incorporate changes gradually and moderately to allow yourself to adjust to the changes, remember it's not a race, it's a lifestyle.

Reality Weight Loss: Page 78

DIETARY TIPS AND TRICKS

Here I'm going to list some tips and tricks that may help you with your weight loss efforts.

Reducing the speed of eating

Here's some tips and tricks that can help you reduce the speed at which you eat. Hopefully with a little bit of humor to help you remember them.

- **Slippery when wet:** Take a drink in between each bite.
- **Starting over:** Set your utensils down in between each bite.
- **Chew-chew train:** Chew each bite thoroughly at least 30 times.
- **Be unique:** Use your eating utensils uniquely. Examples: Use a spoon to eat meat or a fork to eat peas. (This prevents you from overloading your utensils and forces you to take smaller bites).
- **Be special:** Use specialty utensils such as: chopsticks, two pronged forks, etc.

- **Be a socializer:** Talking in between bites can slow your eating speed. (Don't talk with your mouth full).

- **Single cutter:** When eating items that require cutting, cut and eat each bite separately.

- **Hocus focus:** Some people eat fast without even noticing. You may be able to reduce the speed that you eat, simply by focusing and paying attention to how you eat.

- **Downsize:** Reduce the size of the bites you take.

- **That's like eating a board:** Eat foods that require more chewing.

- **Mini pick-up:** Eat foods that limit the amount you can pick up at one time. An example: soup cannot be piled up on a spoon, it limit's the amount that can be picked up.

- **Wow! That's spicy:** Spice up your food, hot or spicy food can limit the speed at which you can eat them, because you need a cooling off period. As a bonus, spicy food can increase your metabolism for a short period of time.

Reducing the amount you eat

Here are some tips and tricks that may help you reduce the amount you eat.

- **Slow Mo:** Slow down and reduce the speed at which you eat. (See previous list).

- **Waterlogged:** Drink a full glass of water before meals. This can make you feel fuller, which will reduce the amount you eat.

- **Get less, more often:** Eat smaller portions more frequently throughout the day. As mentioned earlier this can reduce hunger, as well as increase metabolism.

- **High density:** Eat low-calorie, high-volume foods at each meal. Examples: lettuce, soups, onions, cabbage, sauerkraut, etc.

- **Control freak:** Some people eat everything that is on their plate. If this is one of your problems, reduce the amount that you put on your plate. Slowly reduce portion sizes for everyday consumption.

- **Becoming a boredom control officer:** Find an activity to replace boredom eating. This does not have to be major, simply something that involves your mind such as: light stretching, reading, etc.

- **Stress less:** Incorporate stress management exercises and techniques in order to reduce stress eating. Examples: relaxation, meditation, light stretching or other light activities.

- **Easy does it:** Slowly eliminate food types or amounts, especially trigger foods.

- **Stop being a lab rat:** Reduce the amounts of highly processed and chemically laden foods that you consume. Some chemicals in highly processed foods can trigger cravings.

- **Hey sweetie:** Reduce or eliminate artificial sweeteners. As we discussed earlier artificial sweeteners can trick your body into thinking it's hungry later in the day.

- **Kick the habit and get on the wagon:** Reduce or eliminate alcohol and nonprescription drug use. These items can cause you to eat larger amounts through various means.

- **What's up Doc:** Speak to your doctor about modifying prescription drug types or amounts. Make sure to ask him if all medications are necessary.

- **That empty feeling:** Slowly eliminate empty calorie foods and drinks. Empty calorie foods and drinks are foods that have high amount of calories with very little or no nutritional value. Examples: soda pop, sugary junk food, etc.

- **Clean it up:** Slowly incorporate more natural and clean foods into your diet.

Dietary fats tips and tricks

Here are some tips and tricks to help you reduce the amount of fat you consume or replace unhealthy fats with healthy fats.

- **You don't have to be a sailor to like olive oil:** Sauté with olive oil instead of butter. Use olive oil instead of vegetable oil in salad dressings and marinades.

- **Can ya?:** Use canola oil when baking.

- **Go nuts:** Use nuts or sunflower seeds on salads instead of bacon bits. Snack on nuts instead of potato chips or processed crackers.

- **Nut butter?:** Use non-Hydrogenated peanut butter or other nut butter spreads on apples, celery, bananas, rice or popcorn cakes, etc.

- **Go green:** Use avocado slices on sandwiches instead of cheese.

- **That's fishy:** Eat fish in place of other meats one to three times a week.

DIETARY AND NUTRITIONAL FREQUENTLY ASKED QUESTIONS

Here are some frequently asked questions and answers about dietary and nutritional concerns. These are questions that I have actually been asked, or that I personally wondered about myself at one time or another.

Are there any foods I should completely eliminate or avoid to lose weight?

Obviously any foods that you are allergic to you should try to eliminate or avoid. Other foods you should try to avoid, limit or eliminate would be trigger foods that you just absolutely cannot get under control. Other foods that you may want to try to avoid or eliminate would be highly processed, chemical laden foods and high calorie low nutrient foods. It will be completely up to you, everything will fit in moderation. It is only when we start to consume in excess that it becomes a problem.

How many calories should I be eating a day to lose weight?

There is no one particular calorie amount that will fit everyone. Remember not to drastically reduce calories, not only will this be hard to maintain, but your body will think it is starving, and will actually start to store more fat. In my opinion the best way to adjust your calories, is slowly and moderately, until you find the proper calorie ratio for you.

Are there specific types of foods I should be eating to lose weight?

Not particularly, it is true that the more natural a food is, the better it will be for you. However, you should eat foods that you enjoy and are capable of continuing for the rest of your life. Remember moderation is the key.

How many meals should I be eating a day?

Once again, every individual is different and unique. The only reason for eating more meals is to control hunger and make weight-loss simpler. You can have anywhere from four to six small complete meals throughout the day or three small meals with light snacks in between, or any other combination. It is completely up to you, whatever makes it easiest and most enjoyable. Remember that the number of meals is not as important for controlling hunger as the amount of time in between meals is. Generally to control hunger you should consume a small portion about every two to four hours.

Do I have to eliminate all carbs or all the fat in my diet in order to lose weight?

Absolutely not. As we discussed earlier, carbohydrates and fat are a necessary part of any diet for a healthy functioning body. You may want to reduce and control the amount of carbs and fat's that you consume, but never try to completely eliminate them from your diet.

Do I need to add a lot of protein to my diet?

As we mentioned earlier, consuming anything in excess can be very unhealthy. Athletes and bodybuilders will need more protein than the average person or people interested in general fitness. You may wish to slightly increase protein, again in moderation, but do not go overboard. Excessive protein can put extra strain on internal body organs such as kidneys, liver, etc.

A general guideline for adults is to try to consume somewhere between .8 - 1 g of protein per kilogram (2.2 pounds) of the <u>lean</u> body weight. Notice the phrase lean body weight not total weight. Lean body weight is your body weight minus fat weight. Example: A person who weighs 200 pounds and has 30% body fat has 60 pounds of fat. (200 x 30% = 60). Using the guideline above you would subtract 60 pounds from 200 leaving you with 140 (200 - 60 = 140). You would divide 140 by 2.2 in order to convert to kg and round up to the nearest whole number which is 64. (140 ÷ 2.2 = 64). Now to determine the daily protein requirements we would multiply 64 by .8 or 1 and again round up. (64 x .8 = 52) (64 x 1 = 64) Therefore an adult who weighs 200 pounds with 30% body fat should be consuming somewhere between 52 and 64 g of protein per day. Children and younger adults who are still growing will require more protein than adults. Also note women should increase protein by 30 g per day when pregnant and 20 g per day during lactation.

ACTIVITY AND EXERCISE CONCERNS

In this section I'm going to try to give you some basic information and ideals to increase your activity and fitness level. If you lead a sedentary lifestyle and think that this may be your most likely weight related issue then this is the section you may want to start with.

Once again you should simplify and customize. Use as many or as few of these tips or techniques listed here as you choose. Use a little just to increase your activity and fill-in your daily lifestyle or create your own personalized weight loss exercise system or workout. It's completely up to you, remember keep it simple and fun.

GENERAL ACTIVITY AND EXERCISE GUIDELINES

There are multiple ways to do everything, you will have to figure out what works for you. Here are some generalized guidelines you may find useful in your quest for weight loss success.

Cardio training guidelines

Cardio training is short for cardiovascular training, it is also known as aerobic training. Cardio training is exercise that you do to burn calories and increase cardio respiratory fitness (this is also known as cardio endurance). The intensity of these exercises is generally based on a percentage of your maximum heart rate (MHR). Maximum heart rate is simply a theoretical base number used to calculate target heart rate for exercise. You should not exercise at your maximum heart rate for very long or very frequently. To calculate your maximum heart rate simply subtract your age from 220 (220 - age = MHR). Example: A 35-year-old person would subtract 35 from 220 and get 185 (220 - 35 = 185). Therefore a 35-year-old person's maximum heart rate (MHR) would be 185.

The percentage of your MHR will depend on the Method of cardio you do. There is basically two methods used to train for cardio: steady-state and intervals. Following is a description of these methods and the percentage range of heart rate maximum that should be used.

Steady-state cardio: This is a low intensity cardio method used to train for a constant and steady length of time, generally between 20 to 45 minutes. The percentage of heart rate range should be 50% to 70% of your maximum heart rate. To figure out the pulse rate range for this method, you multiply your maximum heart rate by .50 and .70 to get the minimum and maximum range of heart beats per minute to train between. (MHR x .50 = minimum beats per minute) (MHR x .70 = maximum beats per minute).

Example: Using our 35-year-old from above we would take his maximum heart rate of 185 and multiply it by .50 and .70 to get the value of 92.5 beats per minute (BPM) and 129.5 beats per minute (BPM) respectively (185 x .50 = 92.5 BPM) (185 x .70 = 129.5 BPM). Therefore a person who is 35 years old wanting to incorporate steady-state cardio should train between the pulse rate range of 92.5 - 129.5 beats per minute.

Another very effective and very simple means of testing whether you are training in the optimal range for steady-state cardio is the talk test. The talk test is simply being able to talk without gasping for air while you are training. You may not feel like talking, but you should be able to carry on a conversation. If you cannot carry on a conversation without gasping for air, you are training to hard for steady-state cardio.

Cardio Intervals: This is a high intensity cardio method used to train for shorter lengths of time generally less than 20 minutes. It involves using a combination of low intensity cardio with brief high intensity burst. Example: Jogging for one minute, then running at a fast pace for one minute, then returning to jogging for one minute, and continuing this for the entire training period. It involves intervals of high intensity moments of work and low intensity moments of recovery. Work and recovery lengths can either be the same or different and each may very through out the training session. Intervals can include combinations of various types of exercises including but not limited to: walking, jogging, running, swimming, cycling, hiking, boxing, kickboxing, heavy bag training, stair running, etc. In short intervals can be used with any cardiovascular exercise that you can think of.

The heart rate range used for this method of training is generally between 75% to 85% of your maximum heart rate (MHR x .75 = minimum beats per minute) (MHR x .85 = maximum beats per minute). Again using our 35-year-old as an example, maximum heart rate 185 multiplied by .75 and .85 gives us the value of 138.75 and 157.25 beats per minute (BPM) respectively. I would also like to note at this time that you can round out the numbers. Therefore a 35 year old who wanted to train with intervals would use a pulse rate range of 138 BPM to 157 BPM during the high intensity phase of the interval training session.

It is important to note that the guidelines for these two methods of cardio are just that guidelines. Anything more than you are doing now will be beneficial. If your sedentary, you may have to moderately work up to the lengths suggested in these guidelines.

Resistance training guidelines

Resistance training is training or exercise where you apply muscular contraction against a resistance either internally or externally, in order to improve muscular strength, muscle size, or strength endurance.

Resistance training is usually done using sets and reps. A rep is short for repetitions, a rep is the full range of motion of one exercise technique, such as lifting and lowering a weight. If you lift and lower a weight six times. You have done six reps.

A set is a number of reputations, performed, one after another without a break. If you perform six reps and stop to rest, that is one set. These sets and reps will be different depending on what you're trying to accomplish. Let's take a closer look at each type of training and the sets and reps for each of them.

Strength training: There is two primary types of strength that is trained for, absolute strength and explosive strength.

- Absolute strength: This is the strength that is applied to overcome a resistance in a controlled manner, with out any momentum. Generally people training for absolute strength will use 4-7 sets of 1-5 reps and resting for 3-5 minutes between sets.

- Explosive strength: This is also sometimes referred to as starting strength. This is a strength that is used to explode through the resistance producing maximum momentum. People training for explosive strength will generally use 3-5 sets of 1-5 reps resting for 3-5 minutes between sets.

Muscle size training: This is also referred to as hypertrophy. This type of training is used to break down the muscles, so that they will become larger after they have recovered. People training for muscle size (hypertrophy), generally use 3-8 sets of 8-12 reps resting for 1-3 minutes between sets.

Strength Endurance training: This is also referred to as anaerobic endurance training. This type of training is used to develop a muscle's lasting strength, where it is under resistance for more than two minutes. This type of training is also used to tone and tighten the muscles. People training in this type of resistance generally use 1-4 sets of 15-20 reps. Rest for this type of training is less than one minute between sets.

The number of sets described above is generally referred to as traditional training. And is generally accomplished by training to technical failure on the last rep of the first group of sets, and then training to momentary muscle failure on the last rep of the last set. This can be done by either using a full body workout 2-3 times a week or using a body part split for 4-6 days a week. The general goal is to train each body part 1-3 times a week.

There are two other types of training that can also be applied to the above by modifying the sets and intensity. These other two types of training are referred to as high intensity training and no limitations training. Let's take a closer look at these other two types of training.

High intensity training: The exercises and rep ranges are the same as above. What changes is you only do one set per muscle group and you train to absolute failure. This training is absolutely grueling. To give you an ideal of how grueling this type of training is, a lot of high intensity advocates like to use this quote " if you have not puked, while doing bicep curls, you have not done high-intensity bicep curls". As a matter of fact, if you visit what is usually referred to as a true high intensity gym, you will usually find a bucket somewhere in the workout area. This bucket as you may have guessed is generally referred to as the puke bucket.

Because this training is of such high intensity, people using this method generally only train each muscle group once every 1-2 weeks, in order to allow for adequate recovery. I have personally used this method in the past with very efficient results. However it is very easy to over-train when using this much intensity. I personally over-trained many times while using this training method, and that is the reason I no longer use it. However, if you are (excuse my language), "a balls-to-the-wall" type of person who likes to " get in, get it done and get out" you may want to experiment with this type of training.

Before we move on to the next training type, I would like to clarify the types of failure that we discussed above.

- Technical failure: This is when you can no longer complete an exercise with proper form. Example: your tempo slows down, you start to shake or strain under the resistance.

- Momentary muscle failure: This is when you are no longer capable of lifting the weight, even with strain or improper form, without first resting. After reaching momentary muscle failure, a brief rest will allow you to again lift the same weight.

- Absolute failure: This is when your muscles completely fatigue and you are no longer capable of lifting the same weight, generally for the rest of the day. Example: You lift a weight until you can no longer lift it, then you either use assistance or strip weight off until you can continue lifting, you continue this until you cannot even lift your own arms, even without resistance, this is absolute failure. Generally, the only people who try to reach this type of failure is high intensity advocates.

Now that you understand the differences between types of failure, let's take a look at the other training type, no limitations training.

No limitations training: This type of training uses the principal of practice rather than working out. When using this type of training you use the same principles of rep ranges as you would with the other training types However, you rarely, if ever train to failure of any kind. The theory of this type of training, is that when you train to failure, you are setting limitations on your mind, that tells your body to fail when you reach a certain point. A saying that no limitations training advocates like to use is " train to failure, train to fail". when using this type of training you can set aside a specific time and use as little as 1 set or any number of sets you choose, the key is not to reach failure. You can also, instead of setting aside specific amoúnt of time, you could do different things throughout the day, as mini exercises or opportunity training. Because of the low intensity and practice affect (opposed to working out) you can train in this method up to 5-6 days a week, however, because of the accumulative affect, it is advised to allow your body to recuperate at least 1-2 days a week.

No limitations training is most beneficial to people who may rely on adrenaline when they use their skills such as: law enforcement officers, security personnel, bounty hunters, people who train for self-defense and everyday general fitness. The theory of this is that when you are faced with a high stress situation, your body will produce a chemical called "adrenaline", adrenaline will allow you to accomplish what you would normally not be able to, under normal circumstances. This is what people are referring to when they talk about the " fight or flight" process. When adrenaline is produced the only thing that limits you, is what your mind perceives it is capable of. If you train to failure, your mind perceives this as your bodies capabilities and limitations. By not training to failure you remove these perceived limitations.

Another theory behind this type of training is that, athletes who know when they're going to have to perform at a specific event, can train to failure, and allow adequate time for their body to recover, and be able to peak at the time of performance. However, if you are someone who is training for high stress moments such as self-defense situations, then there is no way that you can possibly know a specific time you will need to perform. If you train to failure on Monday, and you get attacked on Tuesday, but you are too sore to defend yourself, then your training has been counterproductive.

I have personally been using no limitations training religiously for the past year, with excellent, real world results. I am a true believer in this type of training. This is a fairly new training method, and there is very little information about it available. I do not have room in this book to go into complete details, but I hope to get more information out about this training method, hopefully in the near future.

Combination training guidelines

Combination training is a training method where you combine resistance (anaerobic) training with cardiovascular (aerobic) training. The two most common methods used for this is circuit training and conditioning training. Let's take a closer look at both of these methods.

Circuit training: This is a training method that combines resistance training with cardiovascular training. This is done by performing a certain number of resistance training exercises back to back without stopping, moving from one exercise to the next. There is no specific cardiovascular exercises done, the cardiovascular training effect simply comes from the constant movement from one resistance exercise to the next, which will keep your heart elevated for a cardiovascular training affect.

The number of exercises per circuit can be any number you choose. You can alternate between as little as 2 exercises and increase the number of circuits you do, or you could move through 20 or more exercises and decrease the number of circuits. The most common number of exercises is generally 5-10 exercises. You can either do one circuit, or you can perform multiple circuits, resting for a brief amount of time between each circuit.

The rest period between each circuit is generally less than one minute, in order to maintain the cardiovascular training effect. This training method is very effective for people who want to train in both areas, but do not have the time for separate workouts. The rep ranges remains the same depending on what you would most like to improve. Circuits are generally performed as full body workouts, and are generally performed 1-3 days per week, allowing at least one recovery day between workouts.

The resistance training exercises can be any exercise you choose. In order to continue to move from one exercise to the other, you generally perform exercises that alternate muscle groups that are used for each exercise.

You can use completely unrelated muscle groups, such as performing an upper body exercise, then moving directly to a lower body exercise. An example of this would be doing a chest exercise (such as a bench-press or push-up), then moving to a leg exercise (such as a squat or lunge).

You can also use opposing muscle groups (also known as antagonist), such as using muscle groups of one side of the body then moving directly to an exercise that utilizes muscles on the opposite side of the body. An example of this would be doing a chest exercise (such as a bench-press or push-up) then moving directly to a back exercise (such as a pull-up or a row type exercise).

Conditioning: This is another training method that combines resistance training with cardiovascular training. This is very similar to circuit training where you move from one exercise to the next. The difference is that with conditioning training you utilize both resistance exercises and cardiovascular exercises, and you alternate between the two. Another difference, is that you do not use Specific circuits, instead you generally use one of the two cardiovascular type methods steady-state or intervals, and resting when needed.

To do this type of training you would generally do a resistance training exercise (such as push-ups or squats), then immediately do a cardiovascular exercise (such as sprinting or jogging), then continuing to alternate these exercises or different exercises. It is also important to note that you could start with a cardiovascular exercise then do a resistance exercise, the order in which you do them is not important.

In order to utilize steady-state type of training with this method, you would alternate resistance and cardiovascular exercises, using low to moderate intensity, for the entire duration of the training session. In order to utilize intervals for this training method, you would alternate resistance and cardiovascular exercises, using a combination of high intensity moments, and low to moderate intensity or recovery moments. This type of training is very effective for people who need to condition themselves for specific activities. This type of training is done generally 1-5 days a week, allowing at least two days a week for recovery. This method can be utilized by itself or as supplementation to other training methods.

The exercises used for this training method can be anything you choose, it can be specific to your needs, or generalized, simple and fun. You can combine any cardiovascular exercises you choose such as running, jogging, sprinting, jumping jacks, cycling, swimming, skills training (punching, kicking, jumping, etc), or any other cardiovascular exercise you can think of. You can combine these exercises and alternate between any resistance exercises you also choose such as body weight exercises, resistance tubing, weight training exercises (dumbbells, kettlebells, clubbells, etc.), skills training (climbing, carrying, etc.), or any other resistance training exercise you choose.

Cross-over effect

We discussed earlier the attributes of cardio endurance, strength, hypertrophy and strength endurance. I wanted to mention something very important about this type of training. That is the cross-over affect, no matter which attribute you are training for, there will be a certain amount of cross-over. In spite of popular belief, you cannot completely isolate any one of these attributes. What I mean by this is even if you work out with a rep range, training primarily for strength, there will still be a slight improvement in the other attributes including size, cardiovascular health and strength endurance.

When you focus on one attribute, you can improve it more efficiently and more effectively, by training specifically for it, but it will never be completely isolated. This is a good thing, this actually works for you. A lot of people claim that, when you train for strength, you will lose strength endurance or vice versa, this is simply not true. The cross-over effect allows you to train for different attributes while still maintaining the others.

Let's see if we can't use common sense as an example. If you can do 20 push-ups (which is considered strength endurance), and you start a strength exercise program, lifting heavy weights for five reputations per set, and improve the amount of weight that you can lift for those five reputations, then you have become stronger, but if you retest your push-ups you will find that you have also increased the number of push-ups you can perform. Therefore you have not only increased your strength but also strength endurance. It is also worth noting that this same type of exercise would also improve muscle size and cardiovascular health. You can not completely isolate any attribute, so use this to your advantage, when you wish to change or modify your training.

There is however an exception, when you do extreme distance running, for extended periods of time, such as marathon running, this can cause your body to resort to catabolism. Catabolism (also known as destructive metabolism), is where your body breaks down proteins (primarily muscle) in order to produce enough energy. You may have noticed extreme distance runners are extremely skinny with little muscle mass, yet runners such as sprinters and other shorter distance runners, still maintain some muscle mass and have more muscular physiques. If you want to avoid catabolism, you should avoid extreme long distance running.

Mobility and flexibility guidelines

Mobility and flexibility exercises are training methods used to increase the range of motion (ROM) in which you can move your body. Mobility and flexibility drills or exercises can be utilized as supplementation to other forms of exercises. An example of this would be using mobility and flexibility exercises as warm-ups and cool downs for other types of workouts. Mobility and flexibility drills and exercises can also be utilized as a stand-alone workout or training. An example of this would be utilizing exercise and training methods such as Pilates, yoga, tai chi, or other training methods that utilize mobility and flexibility within them.

Mobility and flexibility are very beneficial to everyone of all ages and all fitness levels and goals. Mobility and flexibility share some of the same principles of range of motion improvement, and they are generally classified together as flexibility. However, they do have slight differences. So let's take a look at the differences between the two.

Flexibility: This generally refers to the most extended position of your range of motion (ROM) without the active involvement of the muscle being stretched. Doing flexibility training generally requires you to completely relax the muscle that is directly being stretched. The most common example of this is when martial artist or gymnast performs splits and hold this position. There is basically two types of flexibility static active flexibility and static passive flexibility. Let's take a closer look at these two types of flexibility.

- Static active flexibility: This refers to the stretching of one muscle using the tension or flexing of the opposing (antagonist) muscle. An example of this, is to hold your arm straight out to the side, then use your back muscles to pull the arm backwards, in order to stretch the chest muscles.

- Static passive flexibility: This refers to the stretching of a muscle or muscle groups without muscle tension from any muscles. What provides the stretching force is the effects of gravity on the body or other external force (such as a partner applying pressure to stretch a muscle). An example of this would be when you set in the floor with one leg extended in front of you, deeply breathing and trying to completely relax, while you bend forward until you slightly achieve a stretched tension in the back of the extended leg, you can continue to relax and allow gravity to pull your upper body forward or down. Another example of this would be to extend your arm out to the side, either supported by a partner or against a door frame, completely relax, and either rotate your body, or have the partner move your arm backwards, until a slight stretched tension is achieved for the chest muscles.

Mobility: This is also referred to as dynamic flexibility. It refers to the movement of full range of motion utilizing muscle tension and/or momentum. An example of this, would be a martial artist practicing to improve the height of his kick, by kicking and slowly increasing the height and stretch. Another example of this would be the slow, methodical and balanced movement used by someone participating in yoga, to move their body through different poses, utilizing tension and flow. Mobility is probably the most beneficial type of flexibility you can have. Not only will it aid athletes for specific movements, and prevent injury, but it is also very beneficial for everyone. Mobility will make every day life activities much easier, simpler and safer to perform.

Lifestyle training guidelines

Lifestyle training is the daily activities within your everyday life. It does not have to involve any specific workouts or exercises, that are set aside at specific times. It includes every and any activity you do through out the day, including work, play, family activities, and anything else.

Not every one has to work out in order to lose weight and become fitter and healthier. Leading an active lifestyle is one of the most beneficial and effective means to become fit and healthy. Moderately increasing small increments of activity into your daily lifestyle can not only increase your health and fitness levels but can also improve your perception of overall life quality.

The activities that you add or increase within your lifestyle should be individualized for you personally. Once again customize, simplify, and personalize. Activities should be simple and fun, activities that are complicated, boring or excruciating, will be extremely difficult to maintain and also add unnecessary stress to your life, which as we mentioned before would be counterproductive. These activities can be anything such as playing with your children, incorporating opportunity training, playing sports with friends and family, the activity ideals is limited only to your imagination. So get creative and have some fun.

Warm-up guidelines

The concept of warming up before training is a very controversial topic. Some people believe that warm-ups are absolutely necessary, to prepare your body for activity and decrease the chance of injury. Other people believe that not only does warm-ups not reduce the chance of injury but they are counterproductive to your training activity, especially if you are training for strength, endurance or self-defense.

Warming up before training can be beneficial. If you are training for a specific event that you know when you will have to perform and also be able to warm up before the event, then there is nothing wrong with incorporating warm-ups into your training. Warm-ups can also be very beneficial for generalized fitness training. Warming up at the beginning of training can increase the body's temperature, loosen you up and prepare your body for more strenuous activity. Just use common sense and don't over do it and make sure your warm-ups are compatible with your chosen activity. Also be sure to treat your warm-up as part of your training session, not as a separate function.

On the contrary warming up is not always absolutely necessary and can be counterproductive. If you train for strength, endurance or some other specific attribute, warm-ups can deplete energy stores and pre-fatigue your muscles and body, which could decrease your ability during training and be counterproductive to your goals. If you're conducting this type of activity you may wish to reduce and limit your warm-ups or completely avoid them. Just use caution and common sense and do not push yourself or your body beyond its limitations.

If you are training for self-defense or some other functional lifestyle activity that may be required to perform without notice, once again warming up before training can be counter productive for these types of activities. If you are attacked or you must perform some activity without notice, you will not be able to warm-up before defending yourself or performing that activity. Therefore, when training for these types of situations or activities, you may wish to avoid warm-ups. You should factor in the reasons for training and train accordingly conditioning your body to respond and perform without a warm-up. Here is some advice about self-defense, which I believe you will agree with. If you find you have time to warm up when you are attacked, use this time to escape. Avoiding or escaping a violent situation will prevent injury more than any warm-up ever could. If you choose not to utilize a warm-up just use caution and common sense and do not push yourself beyond what you are safely capable of doing.

Warming up can help prepare your body for activity. However you should realize warming up will not guarantee that you will not be injured. There is also sometimes that warming up before an activity will not be possible or can be counterproductive by using needed energy stores. When you utilize warm-ups, your body can become conditioned to rely on them.

When you condition your body to rely on warming up before an activity, you can increase the chance of injury when you are not able to warm-up. Therefore, it is also important to note, that if you currently use a warm-up but wish not to, because you're body may be conditioned to rely on it , you should slowly reduce the warm-up gradually over a period of time. Do not just eliminate the warm-up, you must re-train your body to perform activity without relying on a warm-up.

There is no definite right or wrong answer, you must use common sense and do what is most beneficial for you and your training. Using a warm-up or not is a personal choice and it is completely up to you. Warming up before training is one of those aspects that is not always a definite good or bad thing. There are times that warming up is sometimes useful and beneficial and there are other times that it is not beneficial and can also be counterproductive, there is a time and place for everything. Once again just use common sense and make the choice that will most benefit you, your training and your lifestyle.

Cool-down guidelines

Unlike warming up, cooling down after training is absolutely necessary. When you do strenuous activity and then stop without slowing and cooling down the blood can pool in your limbs or trained body parts. This can cause your heart to have to work harder to pump the blood throughout the body in order to oxygenate the body and maintain blood pressure. Stopping suddenly after strenuous activity can cause dizziness, fainting and sometimes serious long-term effects, including in extreme cases heart attacks. Cooling down after strenuous activity, allows the body to gradually transition from an exerted state to a resting state safely. Cooling down also helps remove lactic acid from the body, which can help prevent or reduce cramps and stiffness.

Cooling down does not have to be complicated or excessive. Simply continue to move your body at a slower pace or less strenuous Intensity level. Continue to move your body at the slower pace or lower intensity level, until your body cools down, your heart rate slows to normal, and your breathing also returns to normal. There is no specific type of movement to do, any movement you choose to do is fine. Movement can be simple walking, light ballistic stretching such as swinging the arms or legs (nothing drastic), mobility movements, even light stretching after less strenuous activity or any light movement that will keep blood circulating, but still allow your body to slow and return to it's normal state.

Cooling down is not just for the end of training, it also applies to rest periods during training. During training continue to move in between sets, rest periods and other bouts of activity. Keep the body moving do not just stop and definitely do not sit immediately after stopping.

Cool down durations varies for each individual and depending on the activity and intensity level. As a general guideline it is generally done for periods of

5-10 minutes. Just like everything else, cool down durations will be unique to every one. Once again use common sense and self-awareness, no one knows your body better than you do. Be productive, have fun and stay safe.

Recovery guidelines

Recovery refers to the ability of your body to heal and repair itself from the effects of exercise, training and other activities. Your body does not improve during activity, it only improves after it has recovered from the activity performed. If you do not allow adequate recovery between activities you can become over-trained and your body will not improve.

Even low intensity activities can accumulate and will have a breakdown effect on muscles. This break down effect will continue to happen and can increase the chance of injury, until the muscles have a chance to recover and repair. There is basically two common types of recovery, static recovery and active recovery. Let's take a closer look at these two types of recovery.

Static recovery: This refers to actually resting and relaxing, and not doing any type of extra activity except for your daily lifestyle activities. This may even include meditation and relaxation, where you sit quietly and breath deeply to enhance your relaxation.

Active recovery: This refers to doing light activity. Which would be more activity than your daily lifestyle, but not enough to cause extra stress or break down on or within your body. Generally, this is activity that will help you relax such as slow normal walking, light non-dynamic stretching or some other relaxing activity.

As a general guideline it is a good ideal to have at least one static recovery day and one active recovery day per week, if you are new to training you may require more. Also if you are very muscular you may require more recovery time. Larger muscles will take longer to repair than smaller muscles, simply because of the size.

TYPES OF ACTIVITIES

As we mentioned earlier there is multiple ways of doing things, there is also multiple equipment types that you can use when doing them. I've separated these activities into three different classifications which are, body weight training, equipment training and lifestyle training. Body weight training is training that you can utilize without any specialized equipment. Equipment training is training that will require some type of equipment. Lifestyle training is training that can be easily incorporated within your daily lifestyle.

The classifications are of no particular importance, I simply separated them into different classifications, for layout purposes and to prevent having one long drawn-out list. Some of these activities could fit into two or all of the classifications, Once again, the classifications are simply for layout purposes. It is also important to mention that these activities listed here are by no means a complete list, these are just some of the most common types of activities to give you an ideal or starting point. It is important to remember that any activity, even if it is not listed here, will be very beneficial. So let's take a look at some of the types of activities you can utilize to improve your overall health and fitness.

Bodyweight training

Bodyweight training is the process of using your body as a portable gym. Body weight training is extremely effective for improving your overall health and fitness. Arguably, in my opinion bodyweight training is also one of the most functional training types you can participate in. People will more than likely, need to be able to move their body in every day life more, than they will need to move external weights. The activities listed here are activities that you can do with just your body, and do not require any type of equipment. Let's take a look at some of the activities that utilize bodyweight training.

Calisthenics: This is where you utilize your body weight as resistance for various different exercises to develop the different types of attributes we discussed earlier. Examples of this is push-ups, pull-ups, bodyweight squats, jumping jacks, crunches, sit-ups or any other exercise that utilizes bodyweight as resistance. Calisthenics is most commonly associated with military physical training (PT) and school physical education(PE) gym classes.

Yoga: For this type of activity, instead of using the more traditional calisthenics type exercises, you instead move your body fluidly through different poses, while coordinating your breathing with your movements, and by utilizing balance and coordination you try to produce a "tense calm" while holding each pose. There is various forms or styles of yoga including Ananda, Anusara, Ashtanga, Bikram, Integral, Iyengar, Kali Ray Tri Yoga, Kripalu, Sivananda, Svaroopa, Viniyoga combination and hybrid styles. (I apologize to any association or person if I have left any style out). The differences in these styles are generally of what the primary focus is such as flow, body alignment, calorie burning, breath control or some other aspect of the training. Like other types of training there is not a single best style of yoga. If you choose to practice yoga, pick a style that suits you. Yoga is most commonly associated with Indian yogis, however it is becoming increasingly popular around the world, especially within the United States.

Pilates: This is very similar in focus to yoga, in the sense that it focuses on breathing, concentration, flexibility, physical and mental control, centering, body alignment and flow. The differences is within the techniques or positions themselves. Pilates primarily concentrates on the muscles of the core. It also has a very significant focus on mental control. The founder once called this system contrology because he believed that his method uses the mind to control the muscles. Pilates is most commonly associated with its founder Joseph Pilates of Germany. This type of training is also becoming increasingly popular throughout the world, especially in the United States.

Tai chi: This is short for Tai Chi Chuan. This is a Chinese martial art that is called an internal martial art, because of its internal focus on creating health within the bodies internal organs. Tai chi is practiced with forms, which is moving the body very slowly through different postures and coordinating the breath with each movement, while maintaining a focused relaxed mind. Tai chi is sometimes referred to as "meditation with movement." Tai chi can be practiced indoors but most practitioners prefer to train outdoors for the calming and meditative effects of being near nature. Even though tai chi is primarily practiced for health and longevity reasons, the postures used within the practice also have a martial, self defense application. Tai chi is most commonly associated, with the practitioners that can commonly be seen practicing these slow, fluid, and graceful movements within parks allover the world.

Fitness kickboxing: This is also sometimes referred to as cardio kickboxing. This is a form of training that utilizes different techniques from various martial arts and self defense systems, and combines them for calorie burning and other fitness benefits. Kickboxing can be considered a form of conditioning, because of its utilization of kicks, punches and sometimes other exercises including calisthenics to elevate the heart rate and maintain the elevation for certain period of time. Kickboxing is very beneficial to cardiovascular fitness, as well as some of the other attributes including strength, power, speed and strength endurance. The most common and well-known kickboxing training system is probably Billy Blank's Tae Bo®, which has become increasingly popular allover the world, within the past several years.

Martial arts training: Martial arts is a traditional form of self defense training that teaches you to use your entire body for self-defense purposes. I cannot possibly list every single martial art style or system available, but for fitness and health improvement all martial arts would be beneficial. Even though the primary focus is usually on self-defense techniques, most martial arts training usually includes some types of specific conditioning exercises for health and fitness improvement. Even if it does not have specific conditioning exercises, just the fact of practicing the self-defense techniques themselves can be beneficial to health and fitness improvement. Most martial arts will also include some form of mental training such as meditation, relaxation and/or visualization, which is also very beneficial to health and fitness. Martial arts is probably most associated with movies that either realistically or fictionally depicts the martial art systems or styles within them.

Self-defense training: The health and fitness benefits of self-defense training is exactly the same as we mentioned above in martial arts. The difference between self-defense training and martial arts is, that while martial arts focuses on traditional type of training, self-defense incorporates more modern and realistic type of techniques and training for self-defense. This is probably most commonly associated, at this point in time, with Sergeant Jim Wagner's reality-based program and other reality-based systems.

Mobility training: This is a form of training that utilizes natural body and joint movement including opening, closing, twisting, rotations and various other movements for the purposes of improving range of motion (ROM) under realistic conditions. This type of training generally utilize exercises that incorporate movement through a full range of motion, these exercises are sometimes referred to as mobility drills. This is generally used by people who may not enjoy and want an alternative to yoga, Pilates, tai chi and other forms of training that utilizes mobility. Mobility training can not only improve flexibility but also improve strength and other attributes and teach you to move your body under stress or load. Mobility training can be simple joint movements such as those that would benefit the elderly. Mobility training can also become advanced and include specific mobility drills such as those practiced by elite athletes. Mobility training is most beneficial when it is customized to fit each individual's own needs.

Fitness Boxing: This is also known as pugilism. Boxing is a combat sport were two opponents spar using gloved fist. Fitness boxing utilizes the training aspects of boxing for health and fitness purposes. Boxing requires a tremendous amount of both endurance and explosive strength. Boxing training incorporates non-impact work, impact work and road work. Non-impact work includes training such as bobbing, weaving and punching drills, which does not involve impact, an example of this would be shadowboxing. Impact work involves punching drills where your punching involves impacting a person or item, an example of this would be sparring or heavy-bag work. Road work involves cardiovascular endurance conditioning training primarily in the form of running or jogging, can sometimes incorporate bobbing, weaving and punching drills in combination with running or jogging. Fitness boxing can also incorporate equipment such as jump ropes, sparring pads and heavy-bags (mentioned above). This type of training is most commonly associated with the internationally televised sport of boxing. Boxing is also an Olympic event.

Running: This is a generalized term used to describe such exercises as sprinting and jogging, which are just different speeds and intensities of running. Running is primarily used to train for cardiovascular fitness improvement. Running is one of the oldest forms of exercise known to man. Running can be trained specifically for sports or other occasions such as self-defense escape and marathons, or it can be utilized as a generalized fitness exercise. Running can be trained in multiple ways including but not limited to stationary running, road running, hill running, jogging, sprinting, running drills and various other types of drills or exercises. Running is most commonly associated with childhood activities, school gym classes or sports and other types of sports such as Olympic running.

Self resistance training: This is resistance training where you use one muscle or muscle groups against another muscle or muscle groups to increase strength, hypertrophy or some other fitness attribute. This type of training can be utilized with isometric exercises (see below) were the muscle is held in a static position or it can be used with isotonic exercises where the muscle is moved through a certain or full range of motion. Self resistance training can be used with internal or external resistance.

An example of internal resistance is where you would contract, tense or flex your muscles as hard as you could and either hold this position or move certain body parts through a full range of motion while in this tensed state.

An example of external resistance, would be where you use your left hand to push down on your right wrist to provide resistance, and either curl your right hand up through a full range of motion, or provide enough resistance that the tension remains static where the arm cannot move but contracts against the force. This type of training is most commonly associated with the now famous Charles Atlas fitness system, the mail order system whose ads were notably seen in comic's and magazines, sometimes referring to some type of transformation and the phrase " 97-pound-weakling".

Isometric training: This is a form of resistance training where the joint angle and muscle length remains in a static position and does not change during contraction. To do this type of training you would contract your muscles, at a certain joint angle or position, against an immovable object or resistance. This type of training produces tremendous amounts of strength, but only for that one position, not for a full range of motion. In order for this type of training to be truly beneficial you must train in various joint angles or positions within the full range of motion. This type of training, today is generally used as a supplementation for other types of training. This is also most commonly associated with the famous Charles Atlas' mail order training system.

Equipment training

Equipment training is training that requires some type of specialized piece of equipment or area to be utilized. There is multiple types of equipment available I will list some of the most common here.

Dumbbells/barbells: This is weight training equipment used to develop various fitness attributes, most commonly strength and hypertrophy. Dumbbells are weights of various styles and designs, that consists of a short bar (generally shorter than 12 inches long) with weights on each end. Dumbbells are held separately, with one in each hand. Dumbbells are used to develop unilateral strength and fitness, and develops the stabilizer muscles used to move the weights through a full range of motion and keep them separated.

Barbells are weights of various designs and styles, consisting of a longer bar (usually at least 3 feet or longer), with weights on each end. Barbells are held with both hands for one barbell. Barbells are generally used for basic exercises, which require a lot of strength or focus, and are also used to develop good form when first learning lifting techniques.

Both dumbbells and barbells can be either fixed weights, which are not changeable or adjustable weights, that can be changed to various weights. Dumbbells and barbells are most commonly associated with bodybuilders.

Kettlebells: These are specialized cast-iron weight training equipment, developed in Russia. Kettlebell lifting became a national sport in Russia. In Russia a kettlebell is called a girya, and a practitioner is called a girevik. A kettlebell resembles a cannonball with a handle. Kettlebells are used to develop different fitness attributes, primarily absolute strength, explosive strength, strength endurance, agility, balance and functional strength. Kettlebell exercises can include traditional lifts (usually referred to as grinds), swinging type exercises and explosive or dynamic lifts (such as cleans and snatches). Kettlebells are most commonly associated with the Russian Kettlebell challenge (RKC)® made popular by Pavel Tsatsouline who is a fitness instructor and a nationally ranked Kettlebell competitor in the former Soviet Union. Kettlebells are becoming extremely popular throughout the United States.

Clubbells™: This is weight training equipment, consisting of weighted clubs that have the shape and resemblance of the children's plastic fat baseball bat toy. Clubbells™ are used for Circular Strength Training (CST)™ developed by coach Scott Sonnon. CST™ develops strength through your body's normal movements and ranges of motion. CST™ combines movement, structure and breathing into all of its exercises. A similar type of training has been used for thousands of years in various places including India. This type of training can be utilized to enhance any other type of training, or it can be used as a stand-alone training system. This type of training and equipment is most commonly associated with coach Scott Sonnon who is also known for Flow Fit™ and RMax International.™

Exercise tubing/elastic bands: This is a very flexible, elastic, rubber like resistance training tool. Exercise tubing resembles surgical tubing or the rubber tubing that is used in slingshots. Elastic bands are made out of the same type of material as tubing, but instead of taking the shape of tubes they resemble flat bands. This training equipment is a very inexpensive, effective and portable tool for the training of various fitness attributes. Exercise tubing and elastic bands come in various sizes and resistance levels. These devices can be utilized using traditional type exercises or they can be used to provide resistance for specific movements such as punching and kicking. Exercise tubing and bands are probably most commonly associated with exercise and fitness systems being sold on T.V. infomercials.

Weight machines: This is specially designed weight training equipment, that usually consist of cable and pulley systems attached to a weight stack. Weight machines are used to perform exercises that mimics traditional weight lifting and some body weight training exercises. Weight machines provide a constant resistance throughout the full range of motion, however because of the cable or track system they generally do not develop stabilizer muscles. Weight machines are very beneficial for generalized fitness practitioners and resistance training beginners. Weight machines are most commonly associated with commercial gyms and fitness centers.

Weighted hammers: This is weight training equipment that is used to develop functional and circular type strength. Weighted hammers consist of a handle with a weight at one end, these usually resemble a sledgehammer (in fact sledgehammers are sometimes used for this type of training). Weighted hammers come in various shapes, sizes and weights. These training devices can be used by swinging, lifting or striking other objects (such as tires). Weighted hammers are generally used to develop functional laborer type strength, such as found in lumberjacks and construction workers. Weighted hammers are most commonly associated with strongman competitions and training.

Weighted apparel: This is weight training devices, that come in the form of weighted vest, weighted belts, ankle weights and wrist weights. Weighted apparel is generally utilized to add weight or resistance to bodyweight type of training when the bodyweight does not provide enough resistance by itself. Weighted apparel can come in fixed weight styles, where the weight cannot be changed. Weighted apparel can also come in adjustable styles were the weight can be adjusted in certain increments (generally 1 pound). Weighted vest and weighted belts usually come in weights ranging from 10-

75 pounds. Ankle and wrist weights usually come in weights ranging from 5-15 pounds.

Swimming: This is not a piece of equipment, however it may not be available to everyone therefore could be considered a specialized training area or location. Also water provides external resistance and some people may consider pools a type of training equipment. Swimming is self explanatory, therefore I will be brief and simply state that swimming can be a very beneficial type of training used to develop all fitness attributes.

Cycling: This is also self explanatory, it is simply the pedaling of an actual bicycle outside or the pedaling of a stationary bicycle indoors. There is a various types of cycling training including trail riding, mountain biking, street riding, trick riding, racing and various other training or equipment types.

Treadmills: This is specialized training equipment utilized for running and walking type training conducted indoors and in small spaces. Treadmills come in various shapes and sizes, some are motorized and some are simply moved by the user's momentum. Motorized treadmills generally have speed adjustments and adjustments for incline. Most have some sort of safety function that will shut the machine off if a user falls off.

Stair training: This involves running or walking up a set of steps then back again for a number of circuits. This type of training can be utilized with steady-state cardio or interval training. Not only does this type of training develop cardiovascular health but also greatly strengthens the legs and will also benefit the size and shape of the calf muscles of the lower legs. Stair training can be utilized with any set of stairs or steps, anywhere they are found. There is also a specialized machine called a stair stepper, that can be used in a stationary place.

Lifestyle training

As we mentioned earlier lifestyle training is training that can be easily incorporated into your daily lifestyle. Again, it would be impossible to list every single thing that you could possibly incorporate into your daily lifestyle. So I will concentrate on several generalized areas here just to give you an ideal and help you get started.

Walking: Walking is something every single person does in their daily lifestyle, and most people take it for granted, and never realize the benefits. Walking is also one of the most simplest forms of activities that you can do. Walking is extremely beneficial, and can very easily be the base or foundation of any healthy, fit lifestyle. Walking can not only be used for fitness, but can also be utilized for relaxation and focusing of the mind. Try to increase walking within your everyday lifestyle.

Opportunity training: This is the process of utilizing or creating opportunities within your daily life to add extra activity. Everyone has small moments or opportunities to incorporate extra activities within their lifestyle. I'm not talking about the different times that you would set aside to do a specific workout for a specific amount of time. I'm talking about the brief moments of activity in all of our lives, that are usually missed, simply for convenience. Examples of this include taking the stairs instead of an elevator, parking farther away from your destination and enjoying the walk, instead of trying to find the closest parking spot or walking to get your mail instead of driving. There is multiple opportunities through out your daily life, try to do things in a way that will give you the most benefit, instead of trying to do them in a way that is only convenient. Some people say that "opportunity only knocks once", but when you look at it this way opportunity is always knocking, answer the door, seize the day and take advantage of life.

Mini-workouts: This is very similar to opportunity training above. The difference is that mini-workouts, involve taking advantage of brief moments within our daily lives, in order to do some type of specific training exercise. Some examples of this can include, doing calf raises while standing in line, doing a few kicks or punches when no one is looking or even do a few pull-ups every time you come across something that will support your weight. Mini-workouts can even be incorporated into your daily chores some examples of this can include doing certain exercises (such as curls, rows, presses, etc.) with grocery items (such as a gallon of milk, flour, canned items, etc.) while you are putting them away, you could also do certain exercises with a push lawnmower or a vacuum cleaner, or you can simply try to do these chores faster. These mini-workouts are only limited by your imagination. You would be very surprised at how much extra training you can fit into a day, simply by incorporating mini-workouts into your daily life.

Parkour: This is also sometimes referred to as free running. A person who participates in this style of activity is generally referred to as a Traceur. The reason I listed this under lifestyle training is because that many people consider Parkour a part of their daily lifestyle. Parkour is not just about the flips and other tricks that you see on Internet videos. What you see on the videos is generally referred to as "training for the extremes". A Traceur trains for the extremes in order to be prepared for emergencies and to make everyday movements much easier to perform.

Parkour is about moving the body efficiently, it is about overcoming obstacles in the fastest, most efficient and safest way possible. No matter what your skill level is, you can utilize the principles of Parkour in your every day life. After all, no matter what you're training for, isn't one of your goals, to make your body more efficient? Train safe, train efficiently and have fun.

Family and friend activities: This is simply creating more activity within your fun time. Remember as a child when you could run around for hours without getting tired? Why was this possible? Simple! You were having fun. As we stated before when you do an activity that you enjoy doing and have fun doing, not only is it very beneficial, but it is also very easy to do. Take your children for a bike ride or play the good old fashion childhood game of tag. Next time you get together with your buddies play a game of touch or flag football or if you like it rough stick with the tackle version. Some other examples of family and friend activities can include dodge ball, kickball, volleyball, extreme Simon says, basketball and various other activities which again is only limited by your imagination. So get together with friends or family get active and have some fun.

Self-defense/martial arts: I mentioned these under the body weight training classification. The reason I am mentioning them here is because they're a good example, to point out what I mentioned about these activities being able to fit into more than one classification. Different people have different likes, needs and lifestyles, any one of the activities mentioned earlier, in any of the classifications, may be so important to you, that you may consider it part of your lifestyle, rather than a separate activity.

For many people, myself included, self-defense and/or martial arts is considered part of their daily lifestyle. For this reason if you choose to utilize self-defense or martial arts, it is very important that you pick a style or system that enhances and fits into your lifestyle. If your current style or system requires you to change your beliefs or lifestyle, it may be wise to seek out a different style or system.

Gardening: This is a very important part of many people's lives. Gardening can not only be an activity that provides calm and focus, but it can also be very fitness oriented, especially when it includes such activities as raking, hoeing, digging, tilling, and many other gardening aspects. In short gardening can be a very beneficial part of any active lifestyle. If you enjoy this type of activity be sure to include it into your lifestyle. Not only can you breed and grow, flowering life into plants and flowers, but you can also breed life into your everyday lifestyle and allow it to grow and to flower.

Work related labor: Some people including fitness and medical professionals, very easily look over this and never take it into account. Not only is this very beneficial, but it must also be taken into account when considering other forms of training and recovery. If you are overweight, but have a labor-intensive job, you might want to evaluate diet, stress levels and other areas, before you start to add a lot of exercise.

If you add unnecessary exercise to an already strenuously overworked lifestyle, you could very easily become over-trained, which would be counterproductive. Remember everything fits and everything counts. You need to create a healthy balance between work related, laborious activities and other fitness or lifestyle activities within your daily life.

Household chores: Just like work related labor, household chores also count towards activity. Household chores can include such things as taking out the garbage, mowing the lawn, house cleaning and any other household maintenance chore or honey-do project. Household chores are something that you generally have no choice about, they simply have to be done. So by realizing that there are other benefits such as calorie burning, you can turn a tedious chore into something that's at least tolerable. So instead of constantly dreading the chores you have to do, think of them as extra fitness activities for your active lifestyle. Not only will this allow you to reap the benefits of the activity itself, but it can also decrease the mental stress that you use to associate with it. This in and of itself can be very beneficial to your over all health and fitness.

As you can see there is many types of activities that you can incorporate into a healthy, active lifestyle. This is not even close to being a full list, there is many activities that you can incorporate. You can either incorporate them as specific training, exercise or workouts, or you can incorporate them as just something you do on a regular basis within your overall lifestyle. The activity choices are yours, the times you choose to incorporate them are yours, the way you choose to do them are yours and any other aspect is your choice.

You're in charge, you're in control, your activities and your life, enjoy it to the best of your ability.

GETTING STARTED

When first getting started it can be very overwhelming to know where and how to start. You should keep in mind that there is no single one way to do anything. There is multiple ways for you to incorporate activity into your life. Let's take a look at some concepts that may help you get started.

Keep it simple

Remember, what you do to lose the weight, may be what you have to continue to do, in order to keep the weight off. Pick activities that are simple for you to do and will be simple for you to incorporate within your daily life. Even if you have a specific activity in mind, you may need to modify it in order to make it simpler for you to do or incorporate.

Use moderation

By incorporating activity into your lifestyle moderately, you will be more likely to be able to maintain it. Even if you have a specific activity in mind, you may have to slowly work up to be able to do this activity. Make sure that your body has adequate time to accustom itself to the increase in activity.

Remember walking five days a week, will be more beneficial than forcing yourself to run once a month. Walking five days a week may actually lead to being able to run, moderately increase until you get to the point you want to be.

Customize it

Every activity, exercise, work-out or training you do, should fit your needs, wants, likes, goals and lifestyle. Don't be afraid to modify and customize exercises and activities in order to personalize it for you. Even if you have found a specific workout in a magazine or book, there is nothing wrong with changing or substituting some of the exercises to either make it more enjoyable or more beneficial to you. Here's an example: if a workout tells you to do barbell squats, there is no reason why you can not substitute with body weight squats, one legged squats, dumbbell squats, lunges or any other exercise of your choosing.

Make it fun

Just because you're using an activity to lose weight or to get in better shape, does not mean it has to be excruciating or boring. The more you enjoy an activity, the more likely you are to do it, and continue to do it. Some people say life is not all fun and games, this is probably true, but activity for weight loss can be all fun and games. Activity that you enjoy doing, can create fitness, which will allow you to enjoy other activities. Keep this in mind, participating in fun activities with family and friends, will be much more beneficial, than thinking about forcing yourself to do a workout, ever will.

CREATING BALANCE

As you can hopefully see by now, increasing the activity within your daily life and lifestyle, is not that difficult. You can use non-specific activities or specific training and exercises for specific attributes. The choice is completely up to you. No matter what form of activity you choose to utilize you will have to create a balance between different aspects of your lifestyle and activities.

When talking about lifestyle and activities for weight loss, the term "creating balance", can have various meanings including, creating balance for the amount of activity, creating balance within the muscles of the body itself for either appearance or performance, creating balance for the intensity levels of activities, creating balance between the attributes that are being trained for, and last but not least creating balance between your normal lifestyle activities and your fitness training activities. So let's take a closer look at each of these balancing aspects.

Creating balance for activity amounts

What I'm referring to here is creating a balance between the two extremes of not doing enough activity to produce any benefits and doing too much activitiy that produces over-training and is counterproductive.

So how much activity should you do? As we mentioned earlier most health and fitness professionals recommend a minimum of 30 minutes a day. However, this recommendation is rather deceptive, because you cannot train or do lots of activity seven days a week. You must incorporate recovery days, earlier we recommended at least one static recovery day and one active recovery day per week. So let's take this recommended minimum and convert it per week. 30 minutes times seven days gives us approximately 3 ½ hours of activity per week (30 min. x 7 days = 3 ½ hours). 3 ½ hours of activity per week is a more realistic minimum recommendation.

Some of you may be thinking that 3 ½ hours per week seems very daunting. But before throwing your hands up in disgust, let's apply some of the principles we've learned earlier. You can spread this 3 ½ hours out for 5-6 days per week. But wait a minute you say, what about the recommended two days of recovery? That brings us to the next principle we learned any activity counts, this includes the one day of active recovery. The activity you do for your active recovery will count towards the 3 ½ hours of activity per week. And when I say any activity this also includes any activity within your daily lifestyle which may include physical labor related to work, physical activity produced by doing household chores, activities done with friends and family (including the activities involved in raising children), or any other activity within your daily life.

As you can see we have already most likely reduced the 3 ½ hours per week down to a manageable process. But there is still one principle we have not included. That is that the 3 ½ hours per week does not have to be done all at once. Remember you can break this up into manageable chunks of time, including 5 minutes, 10 minutes or any other length of time you choose. So you can slowly start to incorporate activity periodically throughout the day, until you reach the appropriate amount of activity for you.

Now let's take a closer look at how lifestyle activities may affect your overall fitness activities. If you lead a very sedentary lifestyle which includes very little or no activity and very little or no physical effort at work, then you may very well need to incorporate every bit of or more of the 3 ½ hours of recommended activity into your lifestyle. But by contrast if you already lead an active life or work a physical labor-intensive job, you may not need to add any extra activity. If you are very physically active, but still over weight you may want to evaluate the other areas of weight loss such as dietary concerns, medical concerns or mental concerns such as stress.

Creating balance within the muscles of the body

What I'm referring to here, is creating a balance between the muscles that are acting as prime movers (working muscles) and their antagonist muscles (opposing or opposite muscles), for either appearance purposes to keep the body more symmetrical looking, or for performance purposes to allow the muscles to be more efficient, and/or for safety purposes to prevent or decrease the chances of injury. A lot of people feel that working muscles and their antagonist muscles work against each other, however, the reality is all the muscles of the body work together. Antagonist muscles act as a safety mechanism to prevent the working muscle from pulling to hard or to far.

Understanding the terms of antagonist and prime movers is not important. What is important is understanding the concept of how these muscles work together. To clarify this a little more I'm going to give you an example. During a chest pushing exercise such as a bench press or push-up, the chest muscles are the working muscles (prime movers) and the muscles of the upper back are the opposite or opposing muscles (antagonist). An exercise just opposite of this, such as a upper back pulling exercise such as a row or pull up, the muscles of the upper back become the working muscles or prime movers and the chest muscles become the antagonist or opposing muscles. No matter which version of this you're doing, the working muscle provides the tension and force against the resistance, the antagonist muscles acts as a braking or safety system to prevent the working muscles from pushing to far or too hard and causing injury such as muscle tears, muscle pulls, tendon damage or various other types of injuries.

Here are some samples of unbalanced training, some of these you may have witnessed firsthand. Some people will work what is referred to as "mirror muscles". Mirror muscles are the only muscles you see when you look into a mirror, primarily the front of the body. Another type of unbalanced training is people that train what is called "show muscles". These are muscles that show when you are wearing certain types of clothing such as arms and calves, these people while wearing clothes may appear very muscular and massive because of their big arms, but when they remove their shirt they can appear deformed because of such a little chest and shoulders compared to the big arms. Another type of unbalanced training can occur when someone has a physically labor-intensive job that requires them to work certain parts of their body more than others. As we mentioned earlier not only can this type of imbalance have a negative affect on appearance, but it can also negatively impact performance and increase the chances of injury.

It is very easy for the so-called fitness experts to tell you that you should create a workout that works all of the muscles of the body equally. In theory this sounds good, however in reality you have to factor in the other aspects of your lifestyle. As an example, if you are a person who periodically must bend over and pick up heavy items throughout the day, it would be counterproductive to add a workout that involves the same activity such as deadlifts. Instead it would be much more productive for you to balance out the strength ratio by adding abdominal exercises, in order to help support your back, and create more of a balance within the rest of the core muscles.

You must watch for imbalances within your body and try to correct them before they cause any major problems. It doesn't matter whether you are doing a specific workout or any other lifestyle activity, you should be aware of this and factor in all of your activity that could create imbalances and try to create a more productive balance. Do not be partial to one side of the body or certain muscle groups. This is another good example of why you should keep things simple, if you over complicate it is very easy to lose track and create imbalances within the body.

Creating balance for intensity levels

This refers to creating a balance between intensity levels such as high intensity and low intensity and also balancing out recovery time periods for any type of activity. When I say a balance between high intensity and low intensity I'm not necessarily referring to an in-between intensity level such as moderate or medium intensity. Instead, I am referring to creating balance by utilizing various intensity levels periodically, including high, low and anything in-between.

It is sometimes very productive and fun to work at a high intensity level which allows you to push yourself above a certain comfort zone, as long as you don't constantly push yourself or think that you have to push yourself to the brink of destruction. It is also very productive and fun to sometimes work at a lower intensity level, in order to focus on form or develop a certain skill. You can also use low intensity when you first start a new activity to allow your body to become accustomed to this new activity before increasing the intensity level. Utilizing different levels of intensity can also create variety and prevent you from becoming bored with fitness activities.

It is also very important that no matter what intensity levels you use or activities you're participating in, that you allow adequate recovery time for your body to repair itself. Your body does not adapt and improve during the activity, it only adapts and improves after it has fully recovered from the activity.

The old saying "what does not kill you, will make you stronger" can be applied here. When you participate in certain activities your body breaks down, if you continue the same activity without recovery times, you are slowly killing yourself. In order for your body to survive you must allow it to fully recover from the activity, this will allow it to not only survive but to adapt, overcome and improve. Like most of the other balancing aspects, in order to create the most efficient balance, you must factor in all activity and intensity levels that you do, including everyday lifestyle activities and extra training activities.

Creating balance between attributes

What I'm referring to here is balancing out the attributes of cardio endurance, strength, hypertrophy and strength endurance. I'm not suggesting that you try to create an equal balance between all of these attributes, the ratio of each of these will be affected by needs, wants and other factors affecting an active lifestyle that we will discuss later. What I am suggesting is that you simply do not completely neglect other attributes while training for another. You should try to create a balance that will benefit you and your lifestyle.

As we mentioned earlier, you cannot completely separate these attributes, but when you concentrate on one specific attribute, it will develop and improve much quicker and to a greater degree than the other attributes. You can spend more time training for the attribute that you need and want, but it is sometimes beneficial to periodically train in other attributes for a short period of time. As we mentioned earlier you should not change your training simply for change itself or because someone says you need to change it frequently. But if you become bored with a certain type of training or your body no longer responds efficiently to a certain type of training, you can and should change to a different type of training in order to stay interested and keep your body responding efficiently.

How often you change a training type or how long you continue doing a training type, will be completely up to you, there is no magic time that fits everyone. If you're training for a specific attribute, and you are not bored with the training and that attribute is developing and improving efficiently, then there is no reason why you cannot continue training for that attribute. However, if you become bored, the attribute your training for stops improving efficiently or you feel that another attribute needs to be improved, then you can change and start to train for another attribute.

Try to keep the attributes at a balanced ratio that will benefit your lifestyle and specific needs. Some people will need more endurance, others may need more strength and every individual will have their own unique needs and wants for each attribute. Therefore the balance ratio for these attributes will also be unique to each individual. Just don't neglect any of the attributes to the point that would be counterproductive to your goals and lifestyle.

Creating balance between normal lifestyle activities and fitness training activities

As you can see from the above discussions, your lifestyle will affect almost every other area of the balancing aspects. Lifestyle activities will affect all other activities you choose to do. Therefore lifestyle activities must be factored in when designing, planning or implementing any type of training program or workout. As we discussed earlier, it is not absolutely necessary to have a separate specific workout or training program. One of the best ways to lose weight, get in shape and stay in shape is to have an active lifestyle. All activities should be considered part of your lifestyle and incorporated accordingly. However, there is some people that no matter how hard they try, they will still consider certain activities as being separate from their normal lifestyle.

No matter what you consider the activities to be, it is very important to create an overall balance within your lifestyle In order to have a better quality of life. If something is negatively impacting your life or lifestyle you must either modify it, eliminate it or compensate for it. One of the aspects that can impact your lifestyle is time. It is very easy for some of these so-called "gurus" and "experts", to say things like "everyone has the same amount of time in a day, 24 hours". In theory this sounds good and it's even true to a point. However, in reality no one will be able to utilize their time the exact same way.

Each individual has different obligations and responsibilities that will affect how they can utilize their time within their life. For people that have plenty of extra time, it will be very simple for them to add a workout or specific training time into their lifestyle. For individuals that has very limited free time, it is very important that they incorporate activities as being part of their lifestyle. They can do this by utilizing the principles we discussed earlier such as mini-workouts, opportunity training and other methods to create an active lifestyle and compensate for the lack of time.

Another aspect that should be considered when trying to balance lifestyle activities and fitness activities, is recovery time. Any activity that produces fatigue or breaks down the muscles of the body, whether it is from specific training or not, must be allowed adequate time to recover and repair the body. There is many other aspects that will affect the balancing of lifestyle and training activities, many of which will be unique to each individual.

Do not look at this as being complicated, on the contrary utilize this to simplify your active lifestyle. This is why it is very important to realize there is no one lifestyle or one way of training that will fit everybody. No one will ever know you or your lifestyle, better than you. Evaluate the factors that affect you and utilize and incorporate a balanced ratio between activities that will simplify and be most beneficial to you.

ACTIVITY TIPS AND TRICKS

Here's some tips and tricks to help you increase your activity and calorie burning in your everyday life. Remember small things accumulate and add up over a period of time.

Use fidgeting to burn calories

Fidgeting is sometimes considered nervous or bored movement. You do not have to be nervous or bored to utilize this for extra calorie burning moments within your day. Be advised there may be certain times were fidgeting is not appropriate.

- **Shake a leg:** While sitting at a desk at work or watching TV at home, shaking your leg can increase the calorie burning effects by small increments.

- **Tap, tap, tap:** Tap your hands or pencils whenever there is something to tap on.

- **Be a swinger:** Swing your arms back-and-forth and side-to-side periodically throughout the day. Swing your legs whenever you sit in a spot that your legs do not touch the ground or floor. Not only can these activities create a small increase in calorie burning but they can also help keep your limbs limber and flexible.

Take advantage of opportunity training

Utilize extra effort, training or activity whenever the opportunity presents itself. These opportunities are available through out your daily life, you simply have to pay attention and look for them.

- **Walk the walk:** Park in the farther parking spots and take advantage of the walk, instead of trying to find the closest parking spot for convenience.

- **Become a Stairmaster:** Use the stairs instead of an elevator whenever possible, to burn extra calories.

- **Take the mail or paper route:** For those of you who have a long driveway, walk to get your paper or mail, instead of driving.

- **Loosen up:** When sitting for long periods of time, periodically stretch and move your body to stay loose. You can even sometimes utilize your chair for twisting movements.

- **Skip-to-my-Lou:** When going from one point to another, skip or dance along the way, when no one's looking.

Perform mini-exercises when possible

Do short exercises or training techniques throughout the day, whenever you can. One set of a few reps, will only take a few seconds to a couple of minutes maximum. Not only will this give you extra training and extra calorie burning throughout the day but it could also shorten your regular workout if you perform one. If you pick an exercise that is included in your workout, you could have all of your sets completed before the time of your workout.

- **Don't have a cow!, But do have a calf:** Do calf raises whenever you find yourself standing around waiting.

- **Pull up to the bar:** Do a few pull-ups whenever you come across anything that will support your weight, and allow you to do pull-ups.

- **Sneaky, sneaky:** Do a few kicks, punches or a few reps of any other exercise, whenever no one is looking.

- **It doesn't have to be a lazy boy!:** Tighten your abs and do a few crunches, periodically while sitting in any chair.

- **Go! Speedy! Go!:** Whenever you find yourself walking around or walking from place to place periodically speed up and pick up the pace.
- **Use your flex appeal:** Do iso-tension exercises or flex your muscles

periodically throughout the day.

- **Commercialize it:** Whenever watching TV do some type of exercise during commercials.

- **Meal run:** Navy SEALs run to and from each meal during basic training. Their training is rather extreme and I would not recommend it for the general fitness enthusiast, however you can utilize this concept. Simply do a short sprint or walk before each meal when possible. This does not have to be extreme or long, simply going to the end of your hall and back, or any distance and speed you choose. Not only can these short exercises add up to burn a few extra calories, but it has also been shown that small bouts of exercise can suppress your appetite, making you eat less at each meal.

Utilize family or friend time activities

Whenever you're with family or friends try to do fun activities that will burn extra calories. This can be anything that you can think of, it can be traditional fun and games, or something you completely make up out of the blue. Not only can you burn a great number of calories, but it will also be quality, bonding time spent with family and friends.

- **Tag, your it.:** Play tag with your children or friends. If you think it's childish, use your imagination to customize it to suit your needs.

- **Hey! I didn't say Simon says!:** Play extreme Simon says, utilizing exercises or training techniques.

- **What a bunch of amateurs:** Play some type of sports activity whenever you get together with family and friends. Football, baseball, basketball or any other sport you choose. Customize it to fit you and whoever else is playing, it's your game, play it like you want to play it.

- **Wow! Is that supposed to bend that way?:** Play a game of modified twister utilizing mobility and flexibility exercises and drills.

- **Imagine that!:** Use your imagination and modify existing activities or create completely new ones and try them out. Who knows! You may even invent a new game.

Utilize wake-up movements or training

When you first wake up use small movements, stretches or exercises to help yourself wake-up. It does not have to be drastic or dramatic remember small things add up.

- **Reach for the sky!:** When you get out of bed reach up as high as you can, in order to get a good stretch and help loosen up.

- **Stay grounded:** After getting out of bed, squat down or bend over and touch the floor, then stand back up. Do this as few or as many times as you choose.

- **That's how I roll!:** After waking up do joint rolls or rotations, to help loosen up your joints and prepare them for your daily activities.

- **Crunch time!:** When you first wake up, perform crunches or some other ab exercise before getting out of bed.

- **Get a jumpstart:** Most fitness and health professionals agree that you need 30 minutes of minimum activity per day for a healthy lifestyle. This 30 minutes does not have to be all at once. You can do a short training session before breakfast of 5-10 minutes or any amount of time you choose. Various studies have also shown that training that occurs before breakfast burns primarily fat calories.

- **Hop to it!:** Perform low intensity hops or jumps after getting out of bed, in order to get your blood flowing and prepare your body for Your daily activities.

Utilize bedtime movements or training

This is just the opposite of wake-up movements and training. This type of movement and training is utilized to help calm and relax yourself and prepare your body for sleep.

- **Be a smooth operator:** Coordinate slow, smooth, fluid movements with deep, slow breathing to help calm your body and mind. This does not have to be any specific movements, any slow, smooth, fluid movement you choose to do will be adequate.

- **Be a poser:** You can also use static poses, where you get into some type of comfortable pose and hold it, while you do relaxation breathing. You can use one pose or you can use multiple poses and slowly flow from one pose to the next.

- **Go on a bender:** Slowly bend forward, then slowly raise back up, then slowly bend backwards, and once again slowly return to the start, while also coordinating slow, deep, relaxing breathing throughout the entire process.

- **Slow-mo mobility:** Perform regular mobility exercises such as joint rotations, but instead of doing them at the normal speed, slow them down to a very slow movement, while doing relaxation breathing.

ACTIVITY FREQUENTLY ASKED QUESTIONS

Here are some questions and answers that are frequently asked about activity, exercise and training. Once again, these are questions that either I have been asked or have personally, at one time, wondered myself.

Do I have to lift weights in order to lose weight?

Absolutely not! Weight training can be very beneficial but is not absolutely necessary to lose weight or become healthier. As we discussed throughout the book, there is many forms of activity that you can incorporate in order to lose weight and create an active and healthy lifestyle. There is no specific training that you must do. The most beneficial activities that you can incorporate are those that you enjoy and are willing to do. Even if you specifically want to train for strength, strength endurance or hypertrophy, you do not have to specifically use weights, there is many forms of resistance training that we may or may not have discussed earlier such as bodyweight training, exercise tubing, resistance bands and many other resistance types of training. Research and experiment and try to find what you like and is most beneficial to you.

What type of exercise should I do in order to lose weight and become healthier?

Once again, there is no specific type of exercise or training that you should do. Every individual is unique and will have different needs, wants and other factors, that will affect what they can and should do. One of the most important factors will be what you like to do. If you enjoy an activity, it will be much simpler to do, easier to continue and more beneficial to you than any other activity that you do not enjoy. Quit thinking in terms of what you should do and start thinking in terms of what you want to do.

Do men and women need to do different exercises?

There is no straightforward yes or no answer for this question. This Also may not necessarily be only a gender concern, each individual will have their own goals, and will need to adjust the activity types amounts and other aspects for these goals. If men and women have the same goals, they can use the same exercise. If their goals are different they may need different training. Even if men and women want to participate or train together with a specific exercise or activity, they still may need to adjust the way they train, such as intensity, reps and other aspects of that exercise or activity. Whenever incorporating specific exercises or activities into your lifestyle, each individual should incorporate the exercises and activities that will be most beneficial to them. They will generally have certain exercises or aspects that are the exact same, some that are similar and some that are completely different.

Can sleep affect weight loss?

Absolutely! Sleep is a very beneficial part of any lifestyle. Not getting enough sleep can have a huge, negative impact on your health. It can affect every aspect of your lifestyle and training including but not limited to energy levels, recovery, mood, mental abilities, training improvements, skill development, weight, stress levels and many other aspects. Lack of sleep can be extremely dangerous in extreme cases. Too much sleep can also have a negative impact on your life and can affect some of the same aspects. This is one of those things that you should try to create a balance and not go to extremes one way or the other. The most suggested guidelines is to try to get at least 7-8 hours of sleep per night.

I am a single parent, with very little time and I feel guilty when I exercise for an hour, instead of spending it with my children. Any suggestions?

If you feel guilty every time you train, you are probably not getting the best possible benefits, that you could be. Suggestions would depend on what type of exercises you are doing. But if possible one of the easiest solutions is to include your children into your training activities. Not only will you benefit from the fitness aspects of the activity, but you will also be spending quality time with your children and no longer have to feel guilty.

Although some people say that it is safe, I personally do not suggest having children that have not gone through puberty and that are still growing, doing resistance training with weights. (***Caution:*** it has been shown through various studies that weight training with heavyweights can harden the bones. This may be beneficial to adults, but for children who are still growing it may possibly have a negative affect on their growth). They can utilize movements with their own body weight, since bodyweight movement is a necessary part of any living creature's life including humans, this can not only be fun but very beneficial. If you utilize weight training, they can still be involved in other ways such as helping put away certain equipment, counting reps and sets, helping to motivate you and various other ways.

If you do not do a specific training type then you can incorporate activities that you can do with them such as walking, bike riding, active games and various other activities, this can be very fun and beneficial for all of you.

How many sets and reps should I do?

There is no specific one answer for this question. It will be determined by what type of training you're doing and what attributes you're training for. For reps the guidelines we discussed earlier is 6 or less reps for strength, 8-12 reps for hypertrophy, 15-20 reps for strength endurance and two minutes or more for cardiovascular endurance. Again these are simply guidelines and you may wish to experiment with different reps to determine what works best for you.

As for sets again there is various different opinions for how many sets you should do including no specific set range, one set, two sets, three sets and various sets after that, depending on what style a particular person is training in. In reality, there is no specific set range that will work for every single individual. Let's try to apply some common sense to this. If you start by using three sets, and you do not seem to be getting the most benefit from this, where do you go? Do you drop down to two sets, or go up to four sets? When you start with more than one set, and it does not work you do not know whether to increase sets or decrease sets. Therefore I would suggest starting with one set. If one set does not seem beneficial, then it will be obvious to add another set.

Another reason for starting with one set, is that when people first start to train, their bodies adapt very quickly without a lot of intensity. Therefore when you're first starting out you should utilize this and take advantage of it, in order to get the most benefits for the least amount of effort. Also by starting with one set you are allowing your body to become accustomed to this type of training which will allow it to adjust and not become overwhelmed.

What time should I work out or train?

The correct time to workout or train is when you want to or choose to. There is no magic time to workout or train, there is always going to be plenty of people telling you, that you should work out at a specific time and why. But the reality is that you will get better results if you choose a time that fits you, your schedule and your energy levels.

Some people say to work out in the morning, in order to burn more calories specifically from fat. Others say to work out in the evening, because energy levels ramp-up throughout the day. But, once more in reality certain individuals, are just not morning people and may have better results later in the day. Others wake up feeling energized and ready for activity. In short every individual is unique, and you must find what works best for you. Also keep in mind, there does not have to be a specific set time for your training, you can take advantage of brief opportunities throughout your entire day. The choice is yours and there is no wrong or right time to train.

I work in a feed store and lift 50 pound bags of feed periodically throughout the day. This does not count toward my activity does it?

Yes it does count toward your activity. Especially if you're doing it every day and all day. You must consider this when picking other exercises and for recovery purposes. When lifting 50 pound bags of feed, you are at a minimum, working the muscles of the lower back, the glutes (butt) and the back of the upper legs. If you're using proper form while lifting you may be incorporating all of the upper legs, front and back. If you add extra exercise, you may want to add exercises for the abs and other parts of the body, before adding extra for the muscles that are already worked during your day job.

Every activity counts, especially the more strenuous or intense it is. Every activity must be accounted for when planning other activity and when planning recovery periods. Use daily activity, as part of your active lifestyle and overall training regimen, and use it to shorten specific workouts. When training or working out concentrate on other muscles that are not worked any other time and try to create a balance.

How much activity do I need for a healthy lifestyle?

The general guideline is 30 minutes a day or 3 ½ hours per week, however you want to look at it, is fine. And remember this does not have to be all at once or done at a specific time. It does not have to be spread out equally and it does not have to be done in any kind of order. You can spread it out throughout the day, you can do more activity one day than you do on another. It also does not have to be any specific type of activity, any activity you choose will count towards the 30 minutes a day or 3 ½ hours per week. Live your life, have fun and enjoy what you do.

MENTAL TRAINING CONCERNS

Your mind plays a very important part in everything you do including weight loss and fitness. Your mind is not separate from your body, it is a very important part of your body and therefore should be included into any process if you want the most efficient results. Your mind can aid you in obtaining results in many various ways including mindset (what you believe) and mental exercises (meditation, relaxation and visualization). Your mind can be the determining factor of whether or not something will work for you or not work for you. Your mind can also make something that works for you, work better for you.

In this section we are going to take a look at some of the basic mental training aspects that you can use to improve your success. I am only going to cover basic mental training aspects. For most people this will be more than enough. If you wish to train in more advanced techniques you need to seek out a qualified instructor who is familiar with mental training to guide and educate you. It can be very dangerous to train in advanced mental training techniques (such as internal organ control, energy projection, etc.) without the proper guidance of a qualified professional instructor.

MENTAL TRAINING GENERAL GUIDELINES

As with all other weight-loss aspects mental training must be customized and personalized to fit each individual, in order for it to be the most efficient and most beneficial. Following is some general guidelines that you may find useful in the development of your own personal mental training assessment or program.

Body position

You've probably heard of various body positions such as the full lotus and the half lotus that is generally associated with the meditation positions of Yogis and Buddhist. But contrary to what seems to be the popular belief, there is no magic body position that you have to sit in, in order to do any mental training such as relaxation, visualization or meditation. In fact you don't even have to sit, mental training can be done while sitting, kneeling, lying down or even moving.

Here is a list of some general guidelines that will help you in choosing a position for your mental training.

Comfort: The position you choose should be comfortable enough that it does not cause pain or discomfort, that would cause unnecessary distraction. The position you choose should not be so comfortable that you fall asleep. Choose a position that is comfortable but allows you to stay awake.

Uninhibited Breathing: The position you choose should allow you to keep your spine, neck and head in proper alignment, in order to allow you to freely breathe while keeping your breath unrestricted. The position you choose should allow you to take deep natural breaths without straining or forcing.

Natural: The position you choose should be a natural position for you. You do not have to get into any type of unique position that you have never been in before. A position that you are used to being in will be the most effective without causing unnecessary distraction.

Nonspecific: There is nothing wrong with having a favorite position that you utilize the most or even having a specific position for training a specific benefit such as a lying position while in bed and using relaxation to help you sleep. However, you do not want your mind to associate all mental benefits and skills with a specific position. You should try to have more than one position that you can utilize at different times. Keep in mind that any mental training you do whether it's relaxation, visualization or meditation, will eventually be incorporated into your daily lifestyle.

If you ever find yourself in a stressful situation and need to calm down, you do not want to have to sit on the floor and cross your legs or get into any other specific position, you want to be able to continue what you're doing and calm yourself using breathing, mindset and/or visual images. You will eventually want to be able to use the mental skills that you learn anywhere and anytime, even while moving.

Those are some general guidelines that you should keep in mind while determining which positions will be best for you. Try out and experiment with different positions until you find a few or several that you're comfortable with. Always keep in mind that the skills and benefits your training for will eventually be used in your everyday lifestyle for various different situations and purposes.

Breathing

Like body position there is no magic breathing type or pattern. You can use various types of breathing for various purposes, depending on the type of training you are utilizing or the benefits you wish to receive from this training. Before we look at the common guidelines that all breathing types share, let's take a closer look at some of the different breathing types.

Slow breathing: This type of breathing is generally done for calming, relaxing and/or attention focusing purposes. It is generally done by taking slow, deep and natural breaths, while relaxing the body and mind.

Rapid breathing: This type of breathing is generally done to increase the feeling of being energized or to fire yourself up, when you're feeling overly lethargic or lacking the energy to accomplish certain tasks. This type of breathing is done by taking quick or rapid breaths in and out of the body, as quickly as possible. Some people have stated that this resembles hyperventilation. Even though it may have a similar resemblance, it is very important that you never actually hyperventilate. Hyperventilating could lead to lightheadedness or fainting. This type of training is very effective, especially when combined with visual images.

Power breathing: This type of breathing is generally done to increase lung capacity and/or expand the chest cavity. Some people even claim that power breathing will benefit the entire muscle structure of the body and increase overall fitness levels. This type of breathing is done by taking powerful breaths and by trying to take in the maximum amount of air that you can for each breath.

Each inhalation and exhalation is done forcefully while generating tension in the abdominal, chest and other muscles of the body in order to force all of the air out of the body and again to inhale as much air as possible. Some people confuse this with rapid breathing, however while rapid breathing concentrates on speed, power breathing concentrates on quantity. Power breathing does not have to be done rapidly it can be slow and deliberate, or with various speeds.

Nostril breathing: This type of breathing can be done with one nostril, in order to give one side of the brain more oxygen depending on whether you need a more logical mind frame or a more imaginative mind frame. This type of breathing can also be done with alternating nostrils in order to balance out the logical and imaginative side of the brain and to send more oxygen to both sides of the brain for the purposes of reaching a deeper level of consciousness or enlightenment.

In order to use the single nostril method you would close off one nostril and breathe in and out of the other for a few breaths before returning to normal breathing. To increase logical thinking you would close off the left nostril and breathe through the right. In order to increase random or imaginative thinking you would close off the right nostril and breathe through the left nostril.

To utilize alternate nostril breathing you basically inhale through one nostril, then exhale through the opposite, you then inhale through the same nostril that you just exhaled from, then exhale through the opposite. Here's an example you can follow along with in order to get a clearer picture. Close off the left nostril, breathe in through the right nostril, after you complete the inhalation, open the left nostril, close off the right nostril, and exhale out of the left, after you have completed exhaling, inhale through the left, when inhalation is completed, close off the left, open the right nostril, and exhale out of the right nostril, now you're right back at the starting point, to inhale through the right nostril, continue alternating like this for as few breaths or as many breaths as you choose.

That is some of the breathing types that can be utilized for different purposes. Now let's take a look at some general guidelines for all breathing types.

Deep: This is sometimes referred to as belly breathing. Whenever doing any type of mental training your breathing should be deep and expand your belly. Some exceptions can be made for certain types of rapid breathing. But in general breaths should be deep and take in the air all the way to the belly.

Natural: All breathing types should be natural and flow freely and easily, breathing should never be forced. An exception to this can sometimes be made during certain types of power breathing. But again in general breathing should be unrestricted and uninhibited.

Adequate: When utilizing any type of breathing you should be sure that it provides enough oxygen for your body to function. Never do any type of breathing that makes you feel lightheaded or dizzy from a lack of oxygen or too much oxygen.

Simple: If a breathing type or pattern is complicated and hard to remember, it will not be productive for mental training. As you progress you can utilize and try different breathing types and patterns, but they should not distract you from the original or intended purpose. Simplify or become familiar with a breathing type or pattern before utilizing it as your primary type or pattern.

Those are some of the general guidelines that you should keep in mind while determining a breathing type or pattern. But remember there is nothing magical or mystical about any of the breathing types or patterns. Experiment and try different types of breathing and patterns for different purposes and utilize the ones that are simplest and most beneficial to you.

Eye and eyelid position

As with the other guidelines there is no special position for the eyes or eyelids. However, there is a technique that concerns the position of the eye, that will allow you to reach a deeper level of consciousness much more quickly. If you held your head straight, and slightly looked up with your eyes at approximately a 45° angle (does not have to be exact), while keeping your eyes open, after a very short moment you will start to experience slight eyestrain, at this moment you can relax your eyelids, and you will almost immediately fill yourself go into a deeper level of consciousness. This is the natural eye position that your eyes will be in when you are in the level of consciousness that is just below your normal everyday consciousness level. Utilizing this technique will allow you to reach this level of consciousness much quicker than any other method.

As for eyelid position they should simply be relaxed. For most people in order to fully close their eyes or to fully open their eyes they must have tension within the eyelids. Therefore for most people, in order to fully relax the eyelids, they must completely relax the eyelids and relieve all tension, this will generally result in the eye being neither fully opened nor fully closed. With the eyes relaxed you will not have a full field of vision, but there should be a slight space (generally closer to the bottom) that will allow you to see partial images and light.

Focus

As you've probably already guessed, there is no magical or special aspect of focus. Focus is something that simply allows you to maintain a relaxed concentration and prevents your mind from wandering all over the place and becoming distracted. This can be anything that you choose as long as it works for you. What you choose to focus on can include but is not limited to: a spot on the wall, floor or ceiling, a personal item, a structure or item within the area of training, a visual image, a word, a phrase, a question, a thought, a sound, a color, counting breaths or various other items methods or techniques that allows you to keep a soft relaxed focus.

What ever you choose may or may not be unique to you but it must be efficient and effective for you. Because so many people utilize it, I want to mention certain aspects of counting breaths. Breath counting, like anything else you would use, has the primary purpose of keeping your focus and concentration. It is not about the overall number of breaths you take. In fact as a general guideline you should only count to five and then start over. An example is when you exhale Count one, the next exhale Count two, the next three, continue until you reach five, then start over at one. In the beginning you will find yourself counting to eight, nine, ten and higher, when this happens you know you have lost focus and concentration, and should refocus and start over.

Here are some general guidelines you should keep in mind, that concerns focus.

Simple: Whether it is an item or an image it should be simple and readily available. It should be easy to maintain focus on without any strain or major concentration.

Specific: Again, whether it is an item or image you should associate it with what ever your mental training is focused on. If you're doing a relaxation or calming exercise your focus item or technique should be associated within your mind as calming and/or relaxing. If you're trying to gain more energy or enthusiasm the item, image or technique should be associated within your mind as being exciting or containing energy.

Positive: Whatever you decide to focus on should conjure up positive feelings and thoughts within you, in order to achieve positive results. If you focus on something that is negative, it will produce negative results within your mind and body. You must be aware of not only conscious thoughts and feelings but also subconscious thoughts and feelings. If something is looked up on negatively, by the majority of the people within your life or community, your subconscious mind may also perceive this as being negative, even if you are not consciously aware of this negative feeling or perception.

Training times

There are certain times that you will want your mind to associate with your mental training. Preparing yourself for sleep you will obviously want to be associated with bedtime. Energizing yourself and preparing for the day you may want to associate with waking. But not all mental training has to be done at specific times. Anytime you choose or find yourself able to do them will be adequate. There is no right or wrong time for mental training. Remember you will eventually incorporate some of these basic techniques throughout the day within your everyday life.

Another aspect of time that you may be concerned with, is how long should your mental training sessions last. Once again, the choice is yours there is no magical set time frame that is going to be more beneficial than another. Even short periods lasting only five minutes or less can be very beneficial and effective. If you wish to go for 30 minutes to an hour this is also adequate and is completely your choice. Do not miss out on the benefits of mental training because you're avoiding it because you feel you do not have enough time. Remember you're in charge any time, anywhere, any amount and for any length of time you choose.

Trigger words

Trigger words are words that you can get your mind to associate with certain feelings or mindsets. Once your mind associates a specific word with a specific feeling or mindset, simply saying that word either out loud or to yourself, will trigger a response and bring about that feeling or mindset. These do not have to be only words, you can also use phrases.

In order to associate a word or phrase with a specific feeling or mindset, you will need to obtain the desired feeling or mindset, either through a mental training session or naturally. Once you obtain this feeling or mindset, you want to concentrate on this particular feeling or mindset, take several deep breaths, and while continuing to concentrate on this feeling or mindset, repeat the desired word or phrase over and over. By doing this as often as you choose, your mind will eventually start to associate that feeling or mindset with the word or phrase you have chosen. Here are some general guidelines concerning trigger words or phrases.

Length is personal choice: Some people feel that one syllable words work the best. Some people feel that multiple syllable words works best for them. Other people feel that phrases works best for them. There is no definite right answer, there is multiple ways of doing things. Experiment and try different words and phrases until you determine what works the most efficiently and effectively for you.

Specific: The word or phrase you choose to use must be specifically associated within your mind to a specific feeling or mindset. If the word fire makes you think of something that is energetic, then you would want to use fire as a trigger word when you need to develop energy or excitement, you would not want to use it for relaxation. If the word calm gives you a calm and relaxed feeling, you would want to use the word calm as a trigger word for relaxation and you would not want to use it for increasing energy or excitement. The word or phrase that you choose to use must give you the feeling or mindset that you are trying to achieve.

Nonspecific: Don't worry, I'm not being hypocritical or contradictory here. The word or phrase must be specific to the feeling or mindset. However, the word or phrase itself does not have to be specific. You do not have to use the word calm as the trigger word for relaxation. You can use any word you choose as long as it gives you the feeling or mindset you desire. The trigger words or phrases can be unique and personal, that only mean something to you and no one else. The words or phrases can be in any language, can be real or made up, it does not matter as long as they mean something to you. There are no magic words or phrases, only meaningful ones. The words or phrases you use should mean something to you and conjure up the feelings or mindsets that you desire.

Different: You will need to use different words or phrases for different feelings or mindsets. Remember your mind must associate words and phrases with feelings and mindsets uniquely. You cannot use one word or phrase as a catchall to cover all feelings or mindsets. Utilize multiple words and/or phrases for the different feelings and mindsets you need to achieve throughout your daily life.

Visual imagery

Visual imagery is where you imagine a certain image with the trigger word or phrase and associate it with the feeling or mindset you desire to achieve. This is not an absolute must, but if you use trigger words or phrases in conjunction with visual imagery, it can produce much more effective, stronger and quicker results. The same guidelines that applied to trigger words and phrases, apply to visual imagery.

Improving

Don't expect instant results from mental training. As with all other types of training, you will improve with practice. The more you do it the more you will be able to relax. You will be able to reach a deeper level of consciousness. The more you practice you will be able to reach this level of consciousness much more quickly. The more you practice your visual imagery will improve and become much more vivid and realistic. The more you practice the more comfortable you will become with it and be able to extend the session if you choose to do so. The more you practice the more efficiently your mind will associate any trigger words you use with the feelings you want them associated with. The more you practice, the more easier and more efficiently you will be able to incorporate certain techniques and methods within your everyday lifestyle. And as you improve the benefits and efficiency of your mental training will also improve and become much more apparent and noticeable.

Getting started

No matter which one or combination of mental training you decide to utilize, you should start slow and simple, then incorporate other aspects, as your skill improves. Start your mental training in a quiet and non-distracting area. As your skill improves slowly start to incorporate them into other areas of your life that are not completely quiet and non-distracting. Real life itself is not always quiet and non-distracting, in fact real life can be loud, distracting and chaotic at certain times. It is at these times, that your mental training will be the most useful and beneficial.

MINDSET

Your mindset is your beliefs or way of thinking that affects your attitude. Your mindset determines your attitude, behavior and outlook towards life and everything you do within your life. There is many factors that can influence mindset, but ultimately you choose your own mindset. With this in mind let's take a look at how mindset can affect weight loss and fitness.

Power of the mind

The mind is an extremely powerful tool and effects everything you do, this can work for you or against you. If you truly believe that you cannot do something, you absolutely will not be able to do it, until you can convince yourself that you can. In contrast, if you truly believe that you can do something, almost nothing will be able to stop you from doing it.

Whatever your mind believes, whether it is true or not, will generally become a reality. There is an old saying that is based on truth "if you're told a lie long enough, you will believe it, if you believe a lie long enough, it will become the truth". Here is another saying that recognizes the power of the mind, " the body does what the mind tells it to do".

Unlike your conscious mind, your subconscious mind does not see things as good or bad, it takes in every bit of information available through all of the senses and also simply believes what you tell it. The subconscious mind gathers all information and stores it within the subconscious, even when we are not consciously aware of this information. This is how subliminal programming works. When there is a sound or image present, even though we cannot consciously see or hear it, our conscious mind sees or hears it, processes it and stores it as information. Our subconscious mind does this with everything including all of the senses and our thoughts.

If you constantly tell yourself that you are fat, ugly and/or unfit whether it is true or not, your subconscious mind will believe it and set in motion a process to make it or keep it a reality. Therefore it is extremely important for you to try to eliminate any negative thoughts and to utilize positive thoughts.

Harnessing the power

You have very little direct control over your subconscious mind. However you have complete control over your conscious mind. Your subconscious mind gets a lot of its information from and through your conscious mind and sometimes your conscious mind even acts as a filter for the information that is delivered to your subconscious. Therefore you can indirectly control your subconscious by utilizing positive conscious thoughts. You can take advantage of this and use it in multiple ways, any way you choose should be personalized and customized to fit you and your beliefs. Following, is three different ways that you can use to accomplish this. The techniques that you can use in these three ways is limited only by your imagination.

Current reality: This process involves focusing your thoughts on positive aspects that you already currently possess. Find positive aspects within yourself, it can come from anywhere including overall appearance, appearance of certain body parts, attitude, ability or any other positive aspect that you like and are proud of. Allow yourself to acknowledge these positive aspects and think about them throughout the day, in order to drowned out any negative and unproductive thoughts.

Future goals: This process involves focusing your thoughts on what it will be like once you achieve your goals. Allow yourself to think about what you will feel or look like once you have accomplished what you're trying to accomplish. Also continually use positive thinking to convince yourself that you are completely capable of achieving these goals.

Reverse psychology: This process involves creating a mindset or thinking process, that you have already achieved a certain amount of your goal before you actually do. You must use small increments with in your overall goals. In order for this to be the most efficient, it must be believable. An example of this would be if you want to lose 30 pounds, allow yourself to continually throughout the day, think about how good it feels or how good you look, since you lost 2-5 pounds, even though you have just started and have not actually lost any yet. Another example could be, if you wanted to quit something such as smoking or drinking pop, in order to aid yourself for this, continually think about how much better you feel or how much more convenient it is, since you quit whatever it is you're trying to quit, again even before you have actually quit. This way of thinking can encourage your subconscious mind into putting in motion a process that can help you attain and possibly make your goals easier to achieve.

Mental balance

It is human nature to go from one extreme to the other, the way we think is no exception to this. Some people are what is considered optimist you've probably heard this referred to as "the glass is half full" way of thinking. Other people are what is considered pessimist which is sometimes referred to as "the glass is half empty" way of thinking. As with all other aspects of your life, usually the most beneficial way of doing things is to create a balance between the two extremes this includes your thinking process and attitude.

Just because you can find the bad in everything, does not mean you should. At the same time, just because you can find the good in everything, also does not mean you should. If you constantly have a negative outlook about everything, you will close your mind and possibly miss out, by not trying something that may have been extremely beneficial. If you constantly have an overly positive outlook, you will be trying everything and changing aspects of your life, before you realize the true benefits you may have received from one of these. Try to create a balance and keep an open mind. Don't be skeptical about everything, allow yourself to try and experiment with new things. Don't be naïve or gullible, allow yourself to stick with something long enough to achieve the benefits and don't be changing every time you hear of something new that you think will be better.

RELAXATION

Relaxation is a very simple but yet very beneficial technique that you can utilize to manage stress and improve recovery from strenuous activity. It can also be utilized to help keep yourself calm during stressful situations or to calm yourself down when you become overly excited. Relaxation techniques should be kept simple and unique to each individual's needs. Relaxation can be as simple as simply taking a few breaths in order to help relax and calm your mind and body or it can become much deeper and involve relaxing not only the mind but also every single muscle or body part individually. Let's take a look at some of the types and levels of relaxation that you can utilize to benefit all aspects of your life.

Partial relaxation: This can be utilized when you cannot completely shut out every thought, such as when you must maintain focus or concentration on something you're doing or that is going on around you. In order to do this you simply slow and deepen your breathing and clear your mind of any unnecessary thoughts or images. The only thoughts or images you hold on to are only the ones that relate to or correspond with whatever it is you need to maintain focus or concentration on. This type of relaxation is used throughout the day during everyday life. It can be utilized while driving, walking, light work, standing, sitting or any other position or light activity. This type of relaxation is probably the relaxation technique that people utilize the most often within their daily lives.

Full relaxation: This is usually utilized when you have an area and time that is very peaceful and non-distracting and when you do not have anything that you must focus or concentrate on. This is very useful while lying in bed before sleep, it will not only help you fall asleep, but can also help you get better sleep. It can also be used when you've had a bad day or extremely stressful day that partial relaxation can not handle, by utilizing full relaxation it will help relieve and wash away stresses of an extremely hectic day. It is also very beneficial for increasing and expediting recovery of muscles after and between strenuous activity.

Full relaxation involves slow, deep breathing ,while consciously relaxing each body part. You can start from either the head or the toes the choice is yours and is of no particular importance. You can relax each body part in multiple ways, here are some examples:

- **Tension:** Contract a body part, certain body parts or your entire body as hard as you can and hold this tension for a little bit of time generally 10-30 seconds or just before it becomes uncomfortable, then release the tension and allow your body or body parts to fully relax. If focusing on only one or a few body parts at a time, systematically continue until you have relaxed your entire body.

- **Phrases:** Using the internal voice of your mind, tell yourself that each body part is becoming more and more relaxed. There is no special phrases or words. Use words and phrases such as your body parts are becoming heavy, feel as though they are melting into the surface you're on, feel so light that they feel like they're floating or any other phrases or words that will allow you to relax each body part. Systematically work through each body part in this manner, until your entire body is relaxed.

- **Visual imagery:** Use your mind to create images that your body or body parts are melting, becoming heavy and sinking into the surface that you are on, that they're becoming so light that they are floating above the surface that your on or any other visual images that will help you relax your entire body as completely and thoroughly as you possibly can.

- **Combination:** You can use one, two or all of these methods in any combination or order that you choose. Use what is most simple, useful, effective and most beneficial to you. Relaxation should be a personal experience and there is no right or wrong way, as long as it works.

For full relaxation, after you have fully and completely relaxed your body using one or any combination of the techniques above or any other method you choose, you should continue your slow, deep breathing and completely clear your mind of any thoughts, continue this relaxation with a clear mind and slow, deep breathing for as long as you wish. If you're using it to help you sleep, you can simply allow yourself to fall asleep, you will wake up in the morning feeling more refreshed than you normally would have.

You can see why you should utilize full relaxation only when there is no distractions or dangers around when you're fully relaxed and not aware of what is going on around you. It is also important to mention that although this method generally works best while lying down, you can also use it while sitting or kneeling. Because of the full relaxation of the entire body it will require you to be in a position that is somewhat supported.

Active relaxation: This is usually utilized while you are conducting strenuous activity, such as running, hard labor, defending yourself in a self-defense situation, athletic event, working out or any other moderate or high intensity activity. This type of relaxation is used to keep your body relaxed and eliminate unnecessary tension to allow you to move more freely and uninhibited. Unnecessary tension and tight muscles makes you fight against this tension and your own body, which will cause you to fatigue much quicker and prematurely. It is also used to prevent you from holding your breath (some people hold their breath during strenuous or stressful activities), holding your breath will reduce the amount of oxygen your body receives, and will cause unnecessary tension and also increase speed and amount of fatigue.

Active relaxation is done by controlling the breathing. During the non-active part of an activity, you will slow and deepen your breathing when possible. During the effort part of the activity such as punching or lifting, you will breathe out forcefully trying to force all of the air out of your lungs. This breathing out phase will increase the power that you're able to generate and it will also force you to breathe in (it is natural to be able to hold your breath when your lungs are full, but when your lungs are empty, your body will naturally want to breathe in) allowing you to deliver needed oxygen to the body. (This is why the yell when striking is stressed by so many martial arts instructors). Like partial relaxation, active relaxation requires you to eliminate any unnecessary thoughts or images and focus and concentrate only on the thoughts that is absolutely necessary for you to complete the task at hand.

I would like to mention that if you want to actually see this in action, with someone utilizing active relaxation, one of the best examples I can think of is to watch one of the earlier Steven Seagal movies. You may be able to witness this in action in any of his first five or so movies. (Above The Law, Hard To Kill, etc.) basically his three word title movies. As you watch the fight scenes pay close attention to how relaxed he appears and how he seems to flow freely through each technique, with what seems like effortless control and movement, this is active relaxation. These are some of the best visual examples of active relaxation that I have seen. I would also like to say that this is also a good example of moving meditation, which is very similar in appearance to active relaxation, when it is seen in action. We will discuss moving meditation later in the meditation section.

Natural relaxation: This is not a relaxation process that you achieve through training or any conscious effort. This is the small relaxation moments that occur naturally through out your life. An example that maybe all of you have experienced at one time or another is, when you've had a hectic, stressful day, you have to rush home to complete certain chores, it seems like you have been going nonstop all day, and then when you finally get to sit down and realize that you have completed all of the tasks that you needed to for that day and can finally relax, a calm peaceful feeling washes over you, that feeling is natural relaxation.

Although you can not train for or achieve natural relaxation through any conscious effort, you can utilize these moments to enhance your other relaxation effort's. During these natural relaxation moments, is one of the most effective times to associate a trigger word or phrase with this feeling. When you realize that you're naturally relaxed simply start doing slow, deep breathing, focus on this feeling, and start to repeat your desired trigger word or phrase, while continuing to focus completely on this natural relaxed feeling. Your mind will eventually start to associate this word or phrase with this feeling. Also by focusing on this feeling when it occurs, will allow you to remember what it feels like and you will be able to achieve it much quicker and more efficiently when using other types of relaxation.

Those are some of the basic concepts of and ways you can utilize relaxation. As with everything else no one is going to force you to do it, if you choose not to. It may not be an absolute must, but in my opinion it is one of the most under appreciated techniques available. Even though it is so simple to do, it can be just as beneficial and effective or even more so than diet or activity. It is extremely effective at aiding your weight loss efforts and overall fitness goals. I strongly recommend incorporating as many of these relaxation types and techniques into your daily life, as much as you possibly can.

VISUALIZATION

We have discussed using visual images for relaxation. Visualization is much more than simply using visual images. It can also be used for much more than relaxation. The uses for visualization is limited only to your imagination. Visualization is about making the visual images as real, as clear and as vivid as you possibly can. It is also about incorporating as many of your senses (sight, hearing, touch, smell and taste), into this process as much as you possibly can. When utilizing visualization you will not simply see images, instead you will live it, and actually be doing it within your mindscape.

Visualization has been proven to develop and improve skills almost as much as actually physically practicing them. By combining visualization and physical practice, skill development and improvement can be twice as effective as doing only one. You can attain the same results or even better results by combining both of these methods for the same length of time that you would normally only train one. In other words, visualizing an activity for 15 minutes and physically practicing for 15 minutes is just as effective as physically practicing for 30 minutes by it's self. Let's take a look at some of the different aspects concerning visualization.

Efficient

You can utilize visualization throughout the day even during certain times that you can not physically train. Some examples of these times include when you're confined in a certain area (such as a small office space or cubicle), when you're injured, sick, lying in bed before sleep, too tired or too exhausted to be able to physically train. Visualization can even be used to aid in skill development before you are actually physically able to perform that skill, making that skill easier and faster to develop, when you are capable of physically performing it.

Visualization can also be very effectively used when you have limited time and must perform shorter training sessions. You could use the time that you have available to physically train, then use visualization to fill in any of the gaps or specifics that you did not have time to physically train.

Visualization can also be very efficient because there is no wasted time. When utilizing visualization you do not have to travel to a specific area (such as a gym or training area), you do not have to set up any specialized equipment and you do not have to wait for a specific time. When you use visualization everything is immediately ready and prepared for you to start training within your mindscape.

Helps make training more effective

Visualization can make all of your training efforts more effective in various ways. By visualizing yourself attaining, achieving or possessing the skills, attributes or goals that you're training for, can help keep you focused on why you are training and help keep you motivated as well as helping you or making it simpler to achieve these benefits.

It has been proven that when you train by just going through the motions, not thinking about what you are doing or why you're doing it, your training is much less effective. By utilizing visualization you can bridge the gap between mind and body, maintaining focus and making every training session much more effective.

Visualization can be utilized before physical training to help you maintain focus and prepare you for what you have to do during physical training. When you first start a training session your mind may not be completely focused and is still focused on thoughts of what has went on within the rest of your day. By utilizing visualization before training you can prepare and focus both your mind and body for training. By eliminating the unnecessary and wasted thoughts and focusing completely on what you're doing, your training will be much more beneficial and effective.

Visualization can be utilized after training to create a mental impression that you have had a flawless training session. When you physically train your body is tired and as your body gets tired your skills lose efficiency with in their form and become sloppy. By visualizing graceful, flawless training after your physical training, your mind will perceive the flawless training as the last activity it has done for that session, your form and technique will be greatly improved by utilizing this method, you will also improve at a much greater rate than you normally would have.

Benefits much more than just skills

Visualization is generally associated with developing and improving skills, however, this is not its only use. Visualization can be utilized in almost every aspect of your life. I cannot possibly list every conceivable way it can be utilized, but I will discuss some of the uses, so that you can get a general idea.

Mindset: You can utilize visualization to help change a mindset, feeling, belief or attitude that you are not satisfied with. If you are sad or angry, you can visualize doing things or being around people that make you happy. If you are overly skeptical about a process or a technique working, for no real or apparent reason, you can visualize the aspects of why it would work, until you convince yourself to give it a fair chance.

Some people have certain negative beliefs that they know are wrong, but have a hard time overcoming them, because of prolonged mental conditioning aspects such as family, friends or personal experiences. These beliefs can take on various forms including but not limited to discrimination (race, gender, age, etc.), fears (heights, relationships, etc.), insecurities (appearance, abilities, self-worth, etc.), and various other forms. By utilizing visualization you can change and overcome these beliefs. In order to do this you will have to use positive beliefs and visualization, about what you know is true, until these positive changes overcome, push out and eliminate the negative beliefs. Because of the prolonged conditioning of these negative beliefs, you cannot expect immediate results. You must use patience and perseverance and continue until you achieve the results you wish. The results and time it takes to achieve these results will be unique and different to each individual, depending on each individual's current beliefs and willingness to change.

Perception: Perception can involve all of the senses of sight, touch, hearing, smell and taste. These perceptions can be real or imagined, either way they will still have an impact on everything you do. How people perceive these senses can greatly affect their weight loss and fitness efforts, either positively or negatively. So let's take a look at some of these sensory perceptions that can affect you and your goals.

Sight perception: This can include body image (whether you perceive yourself to look fat, skinny, lean, muscular, etc.),personal appearance (how you perceive yourself to look in certain clothing while participating in an activity or how you perceive yourself to look while doing the activity itself), training outlook (the perception of how difficult or easy an activity looks), food appearance (the perception of how food looks to you such as savory or unsavory) or any other aspect of sight.

Touch perception: This can include such aspects as training effort (how hard, easy or at what intensity level you perceive an activity to be), pain tolerance (the perception of how much pain, joy, comfort or discomfort an activity causes), dietary touch sensations (the perception of how a food feels in your hands while handling it or in your mouth while chewing or swallowing) or any other aspect involving touch.

Hearing perception: This can include such aspects as activity sounds (how you perceive the different sounds produced during activity such as grunting, moaning, heavy breathing, the beating of an elevated heart, sounds produced by the body or equipment coming into contact with surfaces, etc.), dietary sounds (your perception of the different sounds produced by different foods eaten), hearing ability (the perception of how well or at what level you can hear which can be affected by and during training activity through blood circulation, heat and focus) or any other aspect involving hearing.

Smell perception: This can include aspects such as personal odors (how you perceive smells that is produced by your own body such as sweat), environmental odors (how you perceive smells that you encounter within your training environment), dietary smells (how you perceive the food smells associated with your dietary choices) or any other aspect involving smell.

Taste perception: This can include aspects such as direct taste (the perception of taste of the items you directly place in your mouth such as food), indirect taste (how you perceive taste that is not purposely placed in your mouth such as the salty taste of sweat) or any other aspect involving taste.

As you can see perception can affect every sense and also every aspect of your weight loss efforts including activity and nutritional choices. By utilizing visualization you can either improve, change or heighten your perception of any of these. It is very important to maintain a positive perception for the activities and nutritional choices that you choose.

Self-confidence: This is the self-assurance or belief in your self and the ability that you can succeed. You build greater confidence about doing something each time you do it. By utilizing visualization you can do anything you choose many times inside your mind, you can do it much more than you could if you were to only use physical training. By utilizing visualization you allow yourself to become familiar with the activity and build confidence.

These are only a few of the things that can be improved through visualization. The benefits of visualization are virtually unlimited and can help you not only with your weight loss and fitness efforts, but also in almost every other aspect of your life. Use your imagination, experiment with different visualization techniques and determine different ways for visualization to help you.

First and third-person Point of view

What I am talking about with point of view is how you view yourself or what point of vision you have during visualization training. A first-person point of view is your normal point of view, which allows you to see out of your eyes, you can see your hands and other parts of your body when performing an activity, but you cannot see your entire body. A third person-point of view is the view that you have while watching someone else, which allows you to see their entire body while performing an activity.

There is a lot of controversy over which point of view you should view yourself in while practicing visualization. Some people claim they get better results by using a first-person point of view, which they claim allows them to perceive this as being more realistic and that they are actually doing it. Others claim they get better results from a third-person point of view, which they claim still retains the realism, but also allows them to vary their focus, see and improve things that they would normally not be able to do in any other point of view. There are some people myself included that utilize both points of view at different times, in order to try to take advantage of the benefits of both. Remember everyone is different and there is no right or wrong way to do this. My suggestion to you, is to experiment with both points of view and to either use the one that most benefits you or use both if you feel that both of these points of view has benefits.

Make it as real as possible

The more realistic and vivid your visualization's are the more effective and efficient the results you achieve will be. Use whichever point of view you choose and incorporate as many of your senses as you possibly can. Here is an example that may help give you an ideal.

If you wanted to use visualization to help improve you're ability at doing pull-ups, you would visualize yourself in any point of view you choose. Incorporate the sense of vision by visualizing yourself standing in front of a pull-up bar, you should be able to mentally see different items within the area you chose to visualize including the floor, mats, walls, doors, windows, area outside the windows, the pull-up bar, other training equipment and any other visual images that you can incorporate. You would then start incorporating the other senses. You would feel the surface that you're standing on under your feet, as you grab the bar, you would feel the bar and the pressure of your hands grabbing the bar. You would incorporate the sense of smell, by smelling the different odors and smells, within the area that you're visualizing such as your sweat, the metal and padding of the pull-up bar, the smell of carpet or padding on the surface of the floor, and any other smells you can incorporate. You would incorporate a sense of hearing, by visualizing that you hear the sounds your feet make against the surface of the floor, the sounds that your clothing and body makes when you move, the sound you make when gripping the bar, the sound of your breathing and any other sounds that you can incorporate. You would then incorporate a sense of taste, by tasting the air and the salty taste of your sweat and any other taste that you could incorporate. Once you have incorporated all of these senses you would visualize yourself doing a certain number of pull-ups almost effortlessly, again keeping it within reason and realistic.

It is important to note that when ever you visualize yourself doing something, that you visualize it as being fairly easy or almost effortless. The reason for this is because if you visualize it being difficult or hard this is what your mind will associate and it will become difficult and hard when you actually physically perform it. By making it easy and effortless within your mind, your mind will associate this activity has being easy and effortless, it will then become slightly easier to perform when you actually physically perform it. Remember this will not happen automatically or with only one visualization.

It will take time and will happen gradually, but it will improve your physical ability greatly over time.

The above example may appear very difficult. Do not allow this to discourage you. When you first start the images and visualization's may not be completely real and vivid. You will progress at your own pace, start simple, with what you can do and slowly build and incorporate different senses and more realistic visuals as you progress. When first starting you may only be able to hold one or two images in your mind, but if you use patience and perseverance and continue to practice you will eventually be able to see multiple moving images within your mind. You will eventually become so proficient at your visualization they will appear to be like movies Inside your mind or it will appear that you are actually there personally doing what ever you are visualizing.

Visualization is an extremely beneficial and effective mental training technique. It can be incorporated and effective by itself or it can help lead you into or be incorporated into other mental training techniques. How ever you use it make it your own by personalizing and customizing until it is the most beneficial to you that it can be. You should make it as real as possible but remember even simple visualizations can be very effective.

MEDITATION

Meditation is mental exercises in which you attempt to get beyond the conditioned, "thinking" mind and attain a deeper state of awareness or consciousness. Some people believe that meditation and relaxation is the exact same thing, this however is not true. You can utilize relaxation techniques within your meditation training, but the difference between meditation and relaxation, is your level of awareness.

During relaxation you can be completely unaware of what is going on around you and completely focusing on the calm, relaxed feeling. During meditation you may have the same calm, relaxed feeling, however, you will be completely aware of everything that goes on around you. You will not completely focus on the things that goes on around you or allow them to guide your focus, but you will be aware of them. In fact the more meditation you do the more your awareness will increase. You will start to be aware of things that you were not aware of when you first began. This awareness will involve all of your senses. During meditation you may see, hear, taste, smell or feel things that you had not in the past. This is part of the meditation process and purpose, it allows you to not only become more aware of yourself, but also more aware of the world you live in and your place in it.

Meditation is not an exercise that you utilize to block out the thoughts or aspects of your life, including those that may cause you stress. It is instead an exercise that allows you to accept, deal with and control the thoughts and aspects of your life.

Reaching a meditative state

A meditative state is simply a level of consciousness that is deeper, calmer and more focused than a normal everyday conscious level. A normal conscious level is unfocused and sometimes very chaotic allowing random thoughts to distract you. A meditative state is a level of consciousness that allows you to fully control your thoughts and focus. Reaching a meditative state is not difficult or complicated. When you first begin you should start in a quiet, non-distracting place and position. Once you become familiar with this meditative state you will be able to achieve it anywhere, any time, even when you are moving.

Just as with any other skill or activity the more you practice your meditation the more you will improve. With each meditation session you will be able to reach a deeper level of consciousness at a much faster rate and you will be able to choose how deep you take your consciousness.

When you first begin, start in a non-distracting area and position. Focus your mind on anything you choose, as we discussed earlier this can be anything. Breathe deeply, but not forcefully, take a full breath in and let all the air out. After a while you will start to feel a change within your body and mind, generally of a relaxed, calm and focused nature. If random thoughts appear in your mind simply allow them to pass and refocus your mind. Do not try to force the thoughts out of your mind, simply allow them to pass naturally and uninhibited.

Here is a technique that was described to me, that may be helpful for you. Think of your mind as being a pond or lake and think of your thoughts as being clouds. A pond or lake, will reflect the clouds images but will not hold them. When the clouds pass, so do the reflections and images. This is how you should allow your thoughts to pass through your mind. Remember everyone is different and nothing is written in stone, if this helps you to think of it this way, then do so, if it does not help you, then find some other way of thinking about it.

That is all it takes to reach a meditative state. The feeling you get once you have reached this state will be unique and personal to you. Everyone may experience different feelings and sensations. Some people describe it as becoming lightheaded. Some described it as a feeling floating in the air. (this may explain why some books, movies and other media outlets depict people hovering above the ground while meditating). Some people describe it as a feeling of being grounded or connected to the surface they are in contact with. Others described it as a serene, peaceful and tranquil feeling. Meditation is a personal experience and what you experience may not be the same as what others experience.

Here are a few pointers that I would like to share with you that may help you achieve a meditative state. Remember meditation is a personal experience. These suggestions are not absolutely necessary, I am simply sharing them with you, because you may find them helpful or useful.

Eyes: I have mentioned this before, slightly look up for small amount of time, and then just before your eyes start to strain, relax them. Do not close them or try to hold them open, simply allow them to relax to a natural un-tensed position. By doing this, you will immediately achieve a deeper level of consciousness, as soon as you relax your eyes.

Hands: There is various positions that you can place your hands in, and various positions that is recommended by various teachers and instructors. My suggestion, is when you are first beginning, simply put your hands anywhere that is comfortable, that allows you to completely relax them without having to physically hold them in position. Also do not place them in a position that causes strain on any other body part, such as behind the neck or head. Placing your hands behind your neck or head, can cause neck strain, cramps or headaches. Also do not sit on your hands, because this can reduce blood circulation causing them to fall asleep and become uncomfortable.

Tongue: Place your tongue on the roof of your mouth and slightly curl it backwards and away from your teeth. This can help increase saliva production, preventing your mouth from becoming dry. It can also allow your tongue to feel more connected to the body and increase focus.

Breathing: I have mentioned there is various ways to breathing during mental training. When first starting to meditate the general practice is to breathe in through the nose and out through the mouth. Breathing deeply and naturally. There is a slight modification that can be very beneficial. When breathing in through your nose use your throat to pull the air in through the nose. One of the easiest ways to learn this is too slowly start to take air in through your open mouth and then close your mouth, continuing to breathe in, the breathing will remain the same, but the entry point will switch from your mouth to your nose. This generally produces an audible sound, that some people describe as being very similar sounding to the breathing of "Darth Vader" in the "Star Wars" movies. Breathing this way, will increase the amount and quality of the air that you're able to take in naturally. By naturally deepening the breathing, you will be able to reach a deeper meditative state, at a much faster rate.

I hope you find these suggestions useful and beneficial. Once you have reached this state of meditation you can simply continue the same procedures for any length of time you would or you can utilize this meditative state for more specific benefits and purposes. Let's Take a look at some of the different uses for meditation.

Meditation utilization

Although meditation can be utilized to clear, calm and focus the mind, this is not its only use. Meditation can be utilized for or within almost anything within your daily life. Let's take a look at some of the different uses for meditation. Here is a partial list of how meditation can be utilized.

- Calm and focus the mind
- Skill development and improvement
- Energy development and control
- Intuition heightening
- Sensory improvement
- Accelerate healing and recovery
- Search for answers or information within sub-conscious
- Habit changing or control
- Change or control mindset and/or feelings
- Prepare mind and body for an activity
- Develop and increase internal awareness (self-awareness)
- Develop and increase external awareness (everything around you)
- Develop and increase creativity
- Mental programming (self-hypnosis)

- Enlightenment
- Moving meditation

These are some of the ways you can utilize meditation but definitely not all. Uses for meditation is almost infinite and is only limited by your imagination. I am not going to go into detail about all of these uses, but I will give some descriptions of some of the most common ones and the ones that can be directly used to enhance your weight loss and fitness efforts.

Skill development and improvement

This is a process of utilizing meditation to reach a deeper level of consciousness and then using visualization to analyze or mentally practice different aspects of a skill that you wish to develop or improve. This type of mental training can be used by itself, such as when you do not have time, energy or space to physically train. It can also be used in conjunction with physical training.

You can use it before the physical training session, in order to completely focus your mind on what and how you want to train. You can utilize it during physical training to completely focus your attention on form, speed, power or any other aspect of a specific skill. You can also utilize it after a physical training session to analyze the training, to help yourself absorb the knowledge from the training or to end the session with flawless training and technique.

Energy development and control

What I am referring to here is the energy that everything is made up of. This energy is referred to many different terms by many different cultures. Some of these terms include but are not limited to; Chi, Hado, Qi, Ki, Prana or Life force energy, it is sometimes translated as the "Breath of Life". One definition of this is, the primordial energy which is the basis for the universe and everything in it. It is the matrix out of which matter and energy are formed, and is some times referred to as the life force in all living things. I would like to note that there is not one single word in the English language that truly describes this concept. However, for simplicity reasons I am going to simply refer to it as energy. I am not trying to lessen the importance of this concept, it is simply for the purposes of simplifying the reading and writing process of this book.

Everything in the universe is made up of energy. Every physical thing including inanimate objects and every living thing including humans, every nonphysical thing including thoughts and the senses are all made up of energy. The energy within yourself and others can be developed and controlled either directly or indirectly. The development of this energy is generally done for health purposes. It is believed that the energy is stored within your body in a spot that is approximately 2 inches below your navel and inside the lower abdomen, this location is sometimes referred to as the "Dan-tian" in many cultures.

Control of this energy is utilized in various ways including but not limited to healing, self-defense, sensory heightening, energy projection and various other aspects. It is important to note that every single meditation conducted involves this energy in some way or another directly or indirectly, whether you are aware of it or not. Like other forms of energy that you may be more familiar with, life force energy has both positive and negative aspects. When referring to positive and negative aspects I am not talking about good or bad, like other energy it is simply positive or negative both of which is needed, both can be beneficial and should generally be balanced.

By utilizing simple and basic meditations you will become more familiar and gain a better understanding and control of this energy. If you wish to learn more advanced control over this energy, you must seek out a qualified professional who is familiar with this type of training and that can personally guide you. I am not going to go into advanced concepts within this book. I will however give you an example that you can use to experience this energy for yourself.

Stand or sit in a comfortable position, hold your hands out in front of you, elbows bent and by your side, hold your hands in a position that resembles holding a ball. For comparison purposes have someone run their arm between your hands before you start this experiment. Have them remove their arm, then start to bring your mind into a deeper level of consciousness through meditation. Breathe deeply and clear your mind. Once you become relaxed and calm, slowly shift your attention to your hands and visualize energy with in your hands. (there is no specific way to do this, you can visualize holding a ball of energy, a ball of water, a ball of air, water shooting from hand to hand, a laser beam going from hand to hand, lightning bolts going from hand to hand or any other visualization that makes it as real as possible to you).

Once you have achieved this visualization and can actually perceive the sensation of energy within your hands, continue to focus on this aspect and have someone once again place their arm between your hands. The sensations that you may experience may include a tingling sensation, warmth, the sensation of actually holding an object, any other sensation or combination of sensations. What the person that sticks their arm in between your hands may experience can include but is not limited to a sensation of warmth, a tingling sensation, the hair on the arms may stick up like with static electricity, any other sensation or combination of sensations. Congratulations, you have not only experienced the energy within your body but have also performed a small manipulation and control of this energy. Remember that all advanced techniques are based on and developed through simple, basic techniques. Not everything has to be as complicated as people would like you to believe. Keep it simple and basic and progress and develop through your own, unique and personal process.

Sensory heightening

Sensory heightening involves improving the quality of the five senses of sight, touch, hearing, taste and smell. Most people take their senses for granted and never truly utilize them to their best ability or advantage. The senses play an important role in every single thing you do, even when you're not fully aware of it. I believe that the senses gives us the ability of intuition. One of the reasons I believe this, is because when you train to heighten your senses, your intuition also increases, even when you do not directly train for it. Therefore in my way of thinking, common sense tells me there must be a connection.

When I refer to heightening the senses, I am not necessarily talking about actually heightening the senses, but rather training the conscious and subconscious mind to be more aware of the senses. There is a lot of people that would immediately be able to use their senses more efficiently, simply by paying attention to them. Here's an old saying that you may find interesting, I do not know where it came from or who said it or even if I'm saying it correctly, but hopefully you can get the ideal and meaning from it. "It does you no good to look without seeing. It does you no good to sniff without smelling. It does you no good to taste without savoring. It does you no good to listen without hearing. It does you no good to touch without feeling".

The senses affect everything you do within your daily life, more than you may actually realize. In fact, just like people have a dominant hand, making them right or left-handed, you also have a dominant sense. This dominant sense affects your perception and interaction with everything and everyone in your life. Let's take a look at how some of these dominant senses may affect you.

Sight: People whose dominant sense is sight will say and do things that are more visually oriented. They may say things that if actually evaluated might not make sense to someone else. They may say " I see what you're saying". Even though you cannot actually see what someone is saying. When someone is speaking to them they may look or stare at them, even to the point of making the speaker uncomfortable. When a person with the dominant sense of sight is speaking, they may feel as though someone is not listening to them unless the person they are speaking to is looking directly at them.

People with the dominant sense of sight also respond better to visual cues than they do to words. Some visual cues they may respond to are body gestures such as nodding, smiling, frowning, shrugging, thumbs-up or the okay sign hand gesture or various other visual cues that they can actually see. They will generally notice visual things about a person or thing before anything else. They may described people or things as being colorful, bright, drab, dim, beautiful, ugly or some other description that is visually oriented.

These are the same people, who when lying may close their eyes, rub their eyes, put their hands in front of their eyes, hide or touch their eyes in some manner or another, almost as if they believe that if they cannot see the lie, their listener will not be able to see the lie either. People whose dominant sense is sight, will generally use words or phrases that are associated with sight, such as I see, watch, look, see you later, Can I see that, what a sight, I can't believe I'm seeing this, do you see what I'm saying, focus on what you're doing, and various other words, phrases and terms that can be associated with sight.

Hearing: People whose dominant sense is hearing will say and do things that are more auditory oriented. They are more attuned to spoken words and other sounds than they are with any other sensory perception. While being spoken to they may lean forward and slightly turn their head, turning one ear closer to the speaker in order to hear them better. They will generally notice auditory aspects about people and things before noticing anything else. When describing someone or something they may start with phrases or words associated with sound such as saying that someone or something is loud, quiet, soft-spoken, Noisy or any other words, phrases or terms that can be associated with sound.

When lying these people may unconsciously, rub, pull or touch their ear in some way or another, it is as though they are trying not to hear the lie and hoping the listener also does not hear the lie. People whose dominant sense is hearing will generally be more comfortable using words and phrases that are most commonly associated with sound, such as I hear ya, listen, do you hear what I'm saying, I hear that, tune into what you're doing, tune in to what I'm saying, that's music to my ears or any other word, phrase or term that may be associated with sound or hearing.

Smell: People whose dominant sense is smell, will generally say and do things that are more smell oriented. They will generally notice smells and odors more often and more than other people may. While having a conversation with someone they may slightly tilt their head backwards, slightly turning up their nose. (The next time someone turns their nose up at you, they may not be snubbing you or trying to be snobbish, they may be simply trying to pay more attention to you). When trying to describe something or someone they may start with descriptions that are associated with the sense of smell such as saying someone or something smelled good, bad, clean, smelly, fresh or some other descriptor that could be associated with smell.

These are the people who when lying, may scratch, rub, pinch, pull or touch their nose in some way or another, almost as if the smell of the lie was irritating their nose. People whose dominant sense is smell will generally use words or phrases that can be associated with a smell such as do you smell me, I've got your scent now, your sniffing up the wrong tree, something doesn't smell right about that guy, something doesn't smell right about this situation, quit being so fresh or any other word, phrase or term that could be associated with a smell or odor.

Taste: People with a dominant sense of taste will generally say and do things that could most likely be associated with taste. They will generally noticed taste more often and to a greater degree than other people would. When having a conversation with someone, they may consciously or unconsciously, lean slightly forward and slightly open their mouth, almost as if they're trying to taste the words that are being spoken. When describing someone or something they may use descriptors such as salty, sourpuss, sweet, bland or any other descriptors that could be associated with taste.

These are the people who when lying may lick their lips, wipe their mouth, spit or touch their mouth in some way or another, almost as if they're trying to get the bad taste of the lie out of their mouth. People with a dominant sense of taste will frequently use words and phrases such as that leaves a bad taste in your mouth, that looks sweet, you look so tasty, I could just eat you up, he's a salty old fool, you're just an old sourpuss or any other word, phrase or term that might be associated with a sense of taste.

Touch: People with the dominant sense of touch will generally do and say things that is more associated with touch or feel. When having a conversation, they will generally have to touch the person they are communicating with. They may touch their hand or shoulder, they may pat them on the back or stand extremely close, even to the point that it may make the other person uncomfortable. People with the dominant sense of touch will also generally use hand gestures more frequently and more freely than other people. Lots of people use hand gestures when talking, but people with the dominant sense of touch use them more frequently and more prominently. If you was to tie their hands behind their back, they would find it very difficult to communicate.

Similar to people with the dominant sense of sight, people with the dominant sense of touch will also more frequently use body gestures that they can feel rather than words such as, nodding the head, shrugging their shoulders, clapping, giving the thumbs-up or okay sign, smiling, frowning and various other gestures that they are able to feel in some way or another. The difference is within the senses, people with the sense of touch will respond better to gestures that they can actually feel rather than see. These people who when lying may feel it necessary to touch or pick up everything within reach or they may go to the extreme opposite and try to avoid touching everything including their own body, almost as if physical touch will control the outcome of whether the lie is believed or not.

People with the dominant sense of touch will generally use words and phrases such as I feel ya, I'm in touch with that, stay in touch, I'll catch ya later, do you feel what I mean, do you feel me, that must've been rough on you, you make me sick and other words, phrases or terms that could be associated with feeling or touch.

That is some of the different ways that your dominant sense can affect you. It is important to note that just like some people are not considered to be truly right or left-handed, instead they are considered to be ambidextrous, the senses can be very similar. Some people may pay equal attention to two, three, four or even all of their senses, and may not have one sense that is truly dominant.
By learning whether or not you have a dominant sense and what it is, can be very useful for your weight loss efforts. Here are some examples of how you could utilize your dominant sense for activity and nutritional choices.

- If you have a dominant sense of sight, you should try to choose a colorful or visually pleasing area to conduct your fitness activities. You can also try to choose healthy foods that also have bright colors or are visually pleasing in some way or another.

- If your dominant sense is touch you should try to conduct activity while wearing comfortable clothing and perform activities that have a pleasing feel to them. Similarly you can choose healthy foods that have a pleasing feel or texture.

- For the sense of taste you could use flavorful gum or mints before or during activity and only allow yourself this before or during activity. Utilizing the sense of taste for dietary needs should be obvious, simply choose healthy foods that taste good to you.

- If you have a dominant sense of smell you should make sure to wash your clothing after every activity session, so that every time you begin an activity your clothing will smell clean and fresh. You could also use deodorizers or incense in the area that you conduct the activity. Choose nutritional foods that have a pleasing aroma. You can also use air fresheners, incense or cook vanilla within the areas you eat your meals.

- If you have a dominant sense of hearing you could listening to pleasing music while you conduct your activities. You can also utilize this for nutritional purposes by listening to music as you eat. It is important to note that there is no one best kind of music, the music must be pleasing to you. Although some people like to listen to rock 'n roll when working out, if you do not like rock 'n roll this could be counterproductive. Always choose what suits and fits you, according to your taste, beliefs and other aspects.

That is some of the ways you can utilize your dominant sense to help you achieve your weight loss and fitness goals. Use these as only examples, utilize your imagination and create your own ways that will most benefit you.

It is also important to note that although you should utilize certain techniques that is pleasing to your dominant senses, you should not ignore your other senses especially during meditation. Incorporate as many senses as you can within everything you do. When meditating do not focus or force yourself to incorporate a certain number of senses, simply allow yourself to become aware of them with their natural quantity and quality.

In order to heighten your senses you can start with focusing on each sense individually and separately. Pick whichever sense you wish to start with. There is no special order in which you should train them, a good suggestion however, is to start with your dominant sense. You are more familiar and more aware of your dominant sense, which will make this training simpler and easier. Reach a meditative state and then focus entirely on the chosen sense. Try to incorporate every aspect of this one sense that you possibly can. Continue this meditative focus for as long as you wish. After you end this meditation, try to be more aware of this one sense, for the rest of that day and the next. Try to notice and be aware of anything and everything that involves that sense. Wait two to three days and then do the same thing for another sense. Systematically work through all five senses. After you start to become more aware of the senses, you can start to combine them, until you are fully aware of all five senses.

The time that you wait in between training sessions is to allow the mind to fully absorb the training. It does not have to be an exact number of days. A general guideline is at least two days between sessions. If you wanted to you could actually work on one sense per week. Or simply wait 2, 3, 4 or any number of days you choose between sessions.

You can do this type of training periodically whenever and as often as you choose. By doing this type of training you will become more aware of each of your five senses and it will seem as though they have been heightened above their normal capacity. It is also important to note that while training the senses you should not place any judgment on them, simply be aware of them. What I mean by this is do not judge something as having a positive or negative aspect. Do not use mental terms to described them such as pretty, ugly, smelly, rough, smooth, etc. Simply allow yourself to notice and be aware of each of the senses with out any judgmental labeling.

Accelerate the healing process

This is the process of helping your body heal from an injury or recover from training activity much more quickly than you normally would. This can be done by utilizing visualization alone or using a combination of energy control and manipulation with visualization. To use visualization you will achieve a meditative state and then visualize the injury healing or the trained muscles repairing and recovering, you can also visualize the soreness from the trained muscle evaporating like smoke out of the muscle or melting and dripping out of the muscle or any other visualization that helps alleviate the soreness and accelerates the recovery process.

To use energy control and manipulation, you would reach a meditative state and then direct this energy to the injured or recovering area and visualize the energy washing over this area and healing or helping it recover. The actual images or sensory perception you use to symbolize the healing or recovering process is completely up to you, just as long as you associate the process you use with healing and/or recovery. This will not mystically or magically allow your body to heal or recover immediately. It will however speed up the healing and recovery process by a noticeable degree. The effectiveness of this process will be unique to each individual according to their beliefs, focus and abilities.

Habit changing and control

When I talk about habit changing, I'm referring to either the complete elimination of a bad habit or changing or replacing a bad habit with a good habit. What I mean by control, is that not all habits can be considered good or bad, instead they may have positive or negative influences depending on the situation. Habits may be beneficial at certain times but may be inappropriate at other times. An example of this might be the shaking of your legs, this can be beneficial and even allow you to burn an extra bit of calories, but it may not always be appropriate such as during job interviews or other situations. Therefore learning to control these habits can allow you to utilize them when they're beneficial but avoid them during situations that they may not be appropriate.

There is once again different opinions that concern habit changing. Some people believe that you can completely eliminate any habit you wish, if you truly want to. Others believe that you can never completely eliminate a habit, they believe in stead that you can only replace one habit with another. There is evidence that supports both theories. I as well as you may have seen people stop doing certain habits without seemingly picking up any other habit. An example of this could be when someone stops a habit, such as smoking, cold turkey and it never seems to bother or affect them. There is also times that I have witnessed people stop one habit only to pick up another. An example of this is when someone stops the habit, such as smoking, only to develop other habits, such as chewing gum or eating more which causes them to gain weight. Declaring whether one of these theories is the absolute truth is above my education level. Utilizing my opinion and a little common sense I once again be leave that both theories can be true and every individual is unique and will respond differently.

If you believe that you can completely eliminate a habit, that you do not like, then by all means do so. If however you find that it is hard to completely eliminate a habit and you seem to be developing other habits that you do not like, then take a more direct approach and change or replace the habit that you do not like with one that is more acceptable to you. Sometimes it is simply a matter of trial and error. Once again the choice is completely yours, utilize what works best for you.

In order to give you an ideal about how to utilize meditation to eliminate, replace or control habits, let's take a look at some examples.

Habit elimination: Let's say that you have a habit of snacking on a particularly unhealthy item at a certain time during the day. To help yourself eliminate this habit, you could reach a meditative state, then visualize yourself at this time, trying to keep it completely realistic visualizing exactly as you actually do it. But instead of snacking on the food, you would visualize yourself looking at the food and feeling completely satisfied and full with out eating it and no longer wanting it. Utilize this meditation as often as possible. When you find yourself in the actual situation of wanting that snack, focus your mind and think about that satisfied, full feeling that you had meditated about. You will be very surprised at how well this can help you eliminate habits.

Habit replacing: Using the same theme as above, let's say instead of wanting to eliminate the snack, you want to replace it with a healthier snack. One way of doing this would be to reach a meditative state then, once again as realistically as possible, visualizing yourself going for the snack, but once you have visualized yourself seeing the snack, you would then visualize yourself picking a healthier alternative. You would visualize yourself consuming the healthier snack and feeling completely full and satisfied and visualizing that the healthy food tasted better than any other snack you could have had. You would visualize this as often as possible. In reality you would try to consciously make the choice of picking a healthier snack. By combining the two you will be much more likely to replace the unhealthy snack with a healthier choice.

Habit controlling: Slightly modifying the theme above, let's say you are not eating a particularly unhealthy food, but instead you are simply eating too much. Therefore you do not wish to eliminate or replace it instead you simply want to control the amount. One way to do this, would be to reach a meditative state, then as realistically as possible, visualize yourself preparing the snack at a reduced portion size. (If you would normally grab an entire bag of a certain item, visualize yourself only getting a small handful or small number of this item). Continue to visualize yourself consuming only a small portion of the chosen snack and once again visualize yourself feeling completely full and satisfied. Meditate this way as often as possible. In reality make a conscious effort to select smaller portions, and then concentrate on the full and satisfied feeling that you had meditated on.

Those are some examples of how you could eliminate, replace and/or control your habits. There is no specifics, you could utilize this for any habits you wish, and you have to find your own way of doing it. Use meditation and visualization with your own perspective and imagination in order to personalize it and make it the most effective.

Prepare mind and body for activity

By utilizing this you can make any activity safer, more enjoyable, more efficient, more effective, more productive or basically improve the overall quality of any activity you choose. This process is used to eliminate any unnecessary thoughts and bridge the gap between mind and body so that you can completely focus on the goals, the benefits, the purpose and/or the activity itself. It allows you to perform the activity with purpose, rather than simply going through the motions.

To utilize this technique you would reach a meditative state, then clear your mind of any unnecessary thoughts, and focus completely on the aspects of the activity you have chosen. You can focus your mind and thoughts on any aspect such as what you're going to do, how you're going to do it, why you are doing it, how long your going to do it, or any other aspect or combination of aspects that is associated with the activity you have chosen.

You can utilize this technique for any activity not just physical or training activity. You can even use it for dietary activity such as eating or preparing meals. Simply take a small amount of time before meals reach a meditative state and then focus your mind and thoughts on dietary aspects such as what you are going to prepare, how you're going to prepare it, what you're going to eat, how you're going to eat it, how much you're going to eat or any other aspect that may be associated with any dietary activity.

This technique can improve the quality of any activity or function you choose. The practice does not have to be extensive or complicated, it can be very brief and simple. You can achieve many benefits with very little effort.

Mental programming

This is sometimes referred to as self-hypnosis, this process can be utilized to mentally program your mind for various purposes including but not limited to habits, beliefs, attitude, skill development, preferences, healing, recovery, etc. The uses for this process is limited only by your imagination. This process can be done utilizing real-time, internal, mental verbal guidance or it can be done by using external prerecorded audio aids to help guide you through the process. No matter which you choose to use the process is the same. There is also no one right or wrong way of accomplishing this, you must utilize techniques and aspects that are personal and specific to you, your needs, beliefs and goals.

To utilize mental program you would first reach your normal meditative state. Once this meditative state is reached you would use some type of visual and verbal cues to deepen your level of consciousness even deeper than your normal meditative state. Some people visualize themselves standing at the top of a set of stairs, the general number of steps is usually around ten. At the bottom of the steps is a door leading into a room that is unique and personal to each individual. They will usually visualize stepping down one step with each exhalation of breath, this visualization is meant to represent the deepening of the conscious mind. They allow their consciousness to deepen with each exhalation and step. Once they have reached the bottom of the steps they would visualize opening the door to the room at the bottom and entering. This room represents the deepest level of consciousness you can achieve or that you want to achieve. This room appears anyway and contains anything that each individual wishes. Once inside the room you can mentally program anything you wish.

Once again there is no specific way to utilize this process, you can use anything that allows you to reach a deeper level of consciousness. Instead of utilizing stares you could count backwards from any number you wish. People utilizing this method generally count backwards from 100 but it can be any number you choose. Simply allow your minds consciousness to deepen with each number you count down and coordinate this countdown with your breathing.

Once you have reached the level of consciousness you wish you will need to utilize something that represents this deeper level of consciousness. It can be a room like we described above but it does not have to be, it can be anything you choose including but not limited to an area inside or outside, a room or an entire structure with many rooms or anything you choose. This place can be completely made up within your imagination or it can be an actual place that is easy to visualize. The only guideline is that it should be realistic to you. How this place looks or what it contains is also completely up to you. Once again the only suggestion is to utilize only things that is beneficial to your goals such as photographs, filing cabinets, videos or anything else that may help you with your mental programming.

Throughout the entire mental programming session you should incorporate as many senses as possible. Do not force them but simply allow as many that naturally occur to happen. Try to keep the sensory perceptions neutral. What I mean by this is that your sensory perceptions should not invoke any unnecessary influence. The perception of Smell should not be a bad smell or an overly fragrant smell, it should be a simple neutral fresh smell. Your perception of touch should not be overly rough or smooth once again simply a neutral and natural feeling only for the purposes of realism. This applies for all other senses.

After you have done your mental programming you can remain in this deep level of consciousness for as long as you wish. When you decide to end the session you should bring your consciousness back up gradually. This is not absolutely necessary but is generally more effective and beneficial. To bring your consciousness back up you would simply reverse the process that you used to deepen it.

For example if you used the stair method you would simply go back up the stairs slowly, allowing your consciousness to heighten with each step and breath. Once your consciousness has returned to its normal meditative state you can utilize another technique that will allow you to feel fresh and energized. To do this, once you have returned to the conscious level of your normal meditative state, you would mentally say you're going to count from one to five, and when you reach five you will open your eyes and feel completely fresh and energized. Once again there is no specific usage, any words phrases or visualizations you choose will be appropriate as long as it allows you to feel fresh and energized. You can also apply extra terms or visualization, suggesting that you will sleep very peacefully when you go to bed an awaken completely energized feeling better than you've ever have. These are not absolutely necessary but can be very beneficial. This too is only limited to your imagination, be creative and have fun.

You should keep your mental programming within realistic boundaries. The more realistic and believable your programming is the more efficient and effective it will be. Also you should keep it very simple incorporate as many realistic aspects as you can into your visualization but only within your own ability and in a way that keeps this process simple. It is also important to note that the benefits achieved from this process will be gradual and individual.

You should not expect instant changes or benefits. I believe most of you will be very surprised and pleased at how quickly you do achieve benefits, but it will require more than one session to make a difference, utilize and incorporate patience and practice. It is also important to mention, that although you can utilize mental programming for various different applications, you should not incorporate a lot of them within each session.

Do not overwhelm your mind, this will only decrease the effectiveness. Only focus on one or two aspects at a time. Utilize different mental programming sessions for different applications.

Initially you may need to do a few or several mental programming sessions. You can do these back-to-back for up to five days and then allow two days off for absorption or you can do them every other day. Once you start to see the benefits you will no longer need to do these sessions so frequently, instead you may simply do follow-up or refresher sessions once in a while, such as once a month or once every two months, the exact frequency will be individual and will be something you will have to determine for yourself. Mental programming is extremely beneficial and effective, utilize it to the best of your ability for your own unique purposes.

Self-awareness

Self-awareness can include the aspect of simply being more aware of your physical body (which is what we will cover here) and it can evolve into the aspect of being aware of who you are and the purpose you have in life (which is beyond the scope of this book). Being more aware of your physical body is extremely important. It is important to know the difference between soreness caused by physical activity and pain caused by injury. It is also very beneficial to be able to notice small changes internally or externally that occur with or within your body. This will allow you to be able to know whether a dietary or a physical program is working or not, much more quickly.

It is important to note that although you should strive to become more aware of yourself and your body, you should not become so self absorbed that it negatively impacts your life. You should also not become so excessive with different aspects of your body or feelings that you allow yourself to become a hypochondriac and constantly think you are sick in some way or another.

Unlike other meditation exercises during self-awareness meditation you will not try to control any aspect of the exercise. Instead you will simply act as an observer or spectator. To utilize self-awareness exercises, you will achieve a meditative state. Once you have achieved the meditative state, you will simply allow your mind to focus, acknowledge and observe different aspects of your body internally and externally. You can listen to your normal breathing patterns, listen and feel your heart beating, allow yourself to become aware of how your overall physical and mental feelings are. Cover every aspect that you can possibly think of utilizing every sense you can possibly incorporate. The amount of time that you focus on each aspect is completely up to you. The amount of time and the frequency that you spend doing this is also up to you.

Once again this process is only limited to your imagination. Try to become more aware of your body internally and externally and become more aware of your feelings mentally and physically to the highest possible extent you are capable of. Become aware of your normal aches and pains so that you can be aware of changes. The uses for self-awareness is almost limitless. It will allow you to have more control over your diet. It can allow you to receive better benefits from your training activity. It can allow you to be aware of illnesses and injuries sooner than you normally would. It can also increase the overall quality of your daily life.

It is very important that when you are becoming more self-aware that you are completely realistic with yourself. Do not judge yourself negatively or overly positively, simply gather realistic knowledge of yourself and your body. By having self-awareness people have been able to utilize it for various different things. Some elderly can predict a change in the weather simply by noticing a different feeling with their arthritis. Some women know when they are pregnant even before it can be physically or medically detected simply by noticing a slight difference within their body. You can utilize self-awareness for positive aspects by being aware of both positive and negative aspects with and within your body.

Moving meditation

Moving meditation is very similar to moving relaxation. The primary difference is while utilizing relaxation you actually can mentally block out different aspects within your environment, but when utilizing meditation you do not block out any aspects within your environment. When utilizing true meditation your awareness is enhanced and you are completely aware of everything within your environment. Although you are completely aware of everything, you do not focus or make mental judgments about anything except that which is absolutely necessary. Let's look at an example scenario, utilizing different types of mindsets, so that you can get a better understanding about these mental aspects.

Let's say you are walking through a park utilizing an average everyday mindset (not relaxed and not meditative). As you're walking your thoughts may be on what you did earlier today, yesterday or what you're going to do tonight or tomorrow. Your thoughts may be random and un-organized you may be completely unaware of anything that is going on around you. As you walk a squirrel runs up a tree in front of you, you may or may not notice the squirrel. If you do notice, your thoughts may shift to thinking about how cute or funny the squirrel is, then they may drift to what he's doing or to something that is completely unrelated. As you continue to walk through the park, there is a noise coming from the bushes slightly behind you. Once again you may be completely unaware of the noise, but if you do notice the noise your thoughts may turn to fear of thinking it is a mugger or some other dangerous person or animal. If it is something dangerous you may be taken by surprise and injured or worse. If it is not something dangerous your thoughts may be either about what it could have been or how silly you was to think it was something dangerous. You're still physically shaken and upset. You continue on with random thoughts running through your mind still oblivious to anything going on around you.

Now let's look at this same scenario, only this time your mindset is relaxed and in the here and now (but still not meditative). As you walk your mind is relaxed but focused on what you're doing. You do not have any unnecessary thoughts, but you are still not completely aware of everything around you. When the squirrel runs up the tree you again may or may not notice him. If you notice him you may still think that he's cute or funny, but then redirect your mind to the relaxed focus state. When the noise comes from the bushes once again you may or may not notice. If you do notice you would turn face the direction of the noise, your thoughts may wonder if it's something dangerous and what you would do if it was. If it is something dangerous you would not be taken completely by surprise, but your response would still be slowed from the thought process to the action process. If it is not something dangerous you would be extremely relieved and refocus your mind to what you were doing. You would continue on being somewhat aware of what is going on around you but not completely aware of anything.

The last way we are going to look at the scenario is if you was in a meditative mind frame and utilizing moving meditation. As you walk through the park your mind is calm and focused on exactly what is going on at the present time here and now. When the squirrel runs up the tree, you notice and knowledge him but have no specific thoughts toward him. You continue on through the park when you hear the noise in the bushes, you hear it and knowledge it, you turn to face the direction of the noise, but once again do not allow it to direct your thoughts. If it is something dangerous you immediately respond and are more likely to successfully defend yourself. If it is not something dangerous once you acknowledge this, you turn and continue on your path completely aware of everything that is going on around you and what you are doing, but only allowing thoughts that are absolutely necessary about what is going on here and now in the present.

I hope this helps clear up the differences between the different state of consciousness of the mind. To develop the ability to utilize moving meditation, you start normal meditation and slowly start to incorporate movement until you can eventually walk while in a meditative mind frame. You continue to practice different meditations while walking and moving until it eventually becomes natural and you can utilize it in any type of movement or activity you choose. Once again keep it simple, relax, have fun and allow your abilities to develop naturally.

MENTAL TIPS AND TRICKS

Here are some quick tips and tricks that may help you improve, incorporate, accelerate or simplify your mental training exercises.

Be a natural: Use natural feelings and associate them with the mindset and words or phrases to enhance your mental training.

We interrupt our regularly scheduled programming: Utilize mental training mini-sessions during commercial breaks while watching television.

You are getting very sleepy: Use mental calming techniques while in bed to prepare yourself for sleep.

Focus-pocus: Use mental training to increase concentration and focus.

Rage Rover: Use mental training to calm yourself down to prevent road rage.

Power drive: Use mental training to help focus your mind on what you need to focus on, while driving and eliminate distractions.

Be absent-minded once in a while: Every so often use one mental training session to not focus on anything, but instead just allow your mind to empty. Empty your mind and relax for the entire session. This can allow your mind to rest and recover very similar to allowing your body to rest in between activity. This can be done once a week, once a month or anytime you want or feel it is needed.

MENTAL FREQUENTLY ASKED QUESTIONS

Here are some more questions and answers, this time they concern mental training.

Can visualization really help me with weight-loss?

Absolutely! Visualization has been shown to be just as effective as physically practicing something. If you can visualize it, you can achieve it.

How important is mindset to weight loss?

Mindset is one of the most important aspects of anything you do, especially weight loss. It doesn't matter how effective something may be, if you believe it will not work, then it most likely will not. In order for something to work you must believe it will. The more you believe in something the more effective it's going to be. Therefore it is important for you to truly believe and have a positive mindset toward your weight loss goals.

My coach use to say that any sport or activity is 10% physical and 90% mental is this true?

I don't know about the exact percentages, but mental effort will generally be more than physical effort. Let's look at this using a little bit of common sense. You can think about doing something (mental) without actually doing it. But you can very seldom do something (physical) without thinking about it. Therefore mental effort will generally be at least twice the amount as physical effort. Take advantage of this and utilize mental training and aspects as frequently as possible.

Do I have to meditate to get mental benefits?

No. There is many other mental training and exercises that you can utilize that does not involve meditation, such as relaxation, visualization, focus, etc. Meditation is very beneficial and effective for those that choose to utilize it. But you are in charge you can choose to utilize or not to utilize anything you wish. There is many types of mental training and exercises that you can utilize other than meditation. The other forms of mental training and exercises are just as effective and beneficial as meditation.

I heard for meditation or visualization to work you have to do them for an hour or longer. Is this true?

Absolutely not! It has been shown in various studies that short brief mental training exercises can be very effective and beneficial. Just like physical training that does not have to be done all at once or for extended periods of time, mental training can also be done in short intervals throughout the day or anytime you choose, for any length of time you choose. You're the boss, you choose when to start and when to stop.

Is weight loss the only thing I could use mental training for?

Definitely not! The uses for mental training is almost limitless, it is limited only by your imagination. Mental training can be used for skill development, attitude, prayer, enlightenment, extrasensory perception, fear management, business, sports, family life and many other uses to numerous to list in this book. Just listing the uses would probably feel an entire book by itself. Remember there is not just one way to utilize something, experiment for yourself and determine how you can make mental training benefit you and your lifestyle.

To use visualization to help eliminate a food, should I visualize myself eating and not liking the food?

You could, you do not know until you try. This may be the best way for you. However, a lot of people feel that utilizing positive visualizations is more effective than utilizing negative visualizations. Visualizing eating and not liking a food would be considered negative, once again I do not believe in one way of doing things so this may be very effective for you. But if you wish to change it to a positive, you could visualize yourself either feeling full whenever you see that food, or visualize a healthier choice tasting better. Remember, experiment and try it multiple ways until you figure out what works for you.

If I over do mental training will I fall into a deep sleep and never wake up?

Absolutely not! This is the reason that a lot of people avoid doing certain types of mental training such as meditation and deep relaxation, but it is absolutely not true. Even if you fall asleep, you will simply sleep normally and awaken normally just like you would if you had taken a nap. There is no danger of falling into a deep sleep or coma that you cannot awaken from. So stop worrying and start enjoying the benefits.

Isn't meditation a religious practice, and shouldn't it only be done by Buddhist or something?

Many cultures utilize meditation as a religious practice, however, it is not just a religious practice. Anyone can utilize mental training in any way they choose. Remember, there is multiple uses for mental training, many cultures simply believe that meditation increases the effectiveness of prayer. Therefore meditation can be used for prayer, but not, just for prayer, it can be used for anything you choose. Once again, meditation is limited only by your imagination.

I've heard about meditation and it sounds so complicated. How is meditation done?

Meditation does not have to be complicated. To simplify it, look at it as mentally calming your mind and body with the deep natural breathing while keeping your mind focused on something in the present. You can focus on anything including but not limited to breathing, a word, a phrase, an item, a question, a person, a place, a specific spot within the training area or anything you choose. One suggestion concerning what you focus on is to try and pick what has a positive influence on you, in order to get positive results. Continue to focus on your chosen focus point, aspect or item, while breathing naturally and deeply. Allow your body and mind to relax and drop into a deeper level of consciousness. You will mentally and physically feel this change. There is not a specific feeling, everyone's experience will be different and what you feel will be unique to you. Once you experience this deeper level of consciousness and become comfortable with it, you can experiment with different types of meditation for deeper levels of consciousness and different benefits and purposes.

PUTTING IT ALL TOGETHER

No amount of information will do you any good if you do not utilize it and put it into action. In this section I'm going to give you some ideas about how to utilize the information you have just acquired. Once again, these are only ideals, there is multiple ways to utilize this information. It is ultimately up to you, you're in charge, utilize the information in a way that is most efficient and effective for you and your lifestyle.

SELF-EVALUATION

The more you know about yourself the easier it will be to make changes and/or reach goals. You must know what you want to do, what you are willing to do, what you're capable of doing, what you're doing right, what you're doing wrong and anything else that concerns you and your efforts. Simply put, in order to get somewhere, you must know where you have been, where you are at and where you are going.

Analyze or assess

There is basically two ways you can evaluate yourself and your situation, analyzing or assessing. You can use one or both of these methods the choice is yours. To give you better understanding of whether you want to use one or both of these methods lets look at the difference.

Analyze: To analyze something is to gather as much information as possible and thoroughly examine it in great detail in order to learn as much as possible about it. This method generally takes longer and can require several minutes up to an undetermined amount of time.

Assess: To assess something is to take into account only the needed or necessary information, while ignoring the aspects that is not absolutely necessary. This method can generally be done much quicker, taking only a split second up to a few minutes.

If you have a great deal of patience, you may wish to analyze yourself and your situation in order to develop a program or system that is completely suited to you. If you have very little patience, you may wish to do a quick assessment of yourself so that you can get started on a system or program much quicker. You could also utilize both methods by doing a quick assessment of yourself and your situation so that you can start immediately, and then continue to analyze yourself and your situation and fine tune your program or system. Once again, it is completely up to you, only you will be able to determine the best method and what is most efficient and effective for you to utilize.

Determining weight related problems

One of the most important aspects to determine from your self-evaluation, is why you are overweight. Some of you may have one major concern that is the primary cause of your weight problem. Others may have multiple smaller concerns that add up and accumulate to cause your weight problem. Still yet, some of you may have both a major concern that is the primary cause of your weight problem, as well as smaller concerns that add to the situation.

These concerns may be dietary concerns, activity concerns or some combination thereof. Once you have determined what is causing your weight problems, you will be better prepared to take action against them. Try to determine what your biggest or major concerns are and what your littlest or minor concerns are. Take this knowledge and apply it to planning and designing your weight loss program.

DESIGNING AND PLANNING PHASE

Your weight-loss efforts must be part of your lifestyle or at the very least fit into your lifestyle. No matter which perception you take with your weight-loss efforts, the fact remains that your weight-loss efforts will affect your lifestyle and your lifestyle will affect your weight-loss efforts. Therefore your weight-loss efforts and lifestyle must complement and be productive for each other and you must consider this when designing or planning aspects for weight loss.

The degree of planning and designing

How and to what extent you design and plan will be determined by what type of person you are. Remember, you do not have to change who you are, in order to change how you look. If you are a very organized, strict and meticulous person you may wish to design and plan out every detail of your program or lifestyle. In contrast, if you are a very non-organized and spontaneous person, you may wish to plan very little and allow for freedom of choice. Some of you may fall in between these two extremes in which case you would design and plan accordingly. Let's look at these in a little bit more detail so that you have a better understanding and will be more able to determine the best way for you to proceed.

Meticulous: If you're the type of person who is very organized, strict, and meticulous you may wish to plan for every single detail within your life and weight-loss efforts. You may wish to plan every single meal including what you will eat, what time you will eat it and how you will eat it for every day of the week. You may even pick a day that your pre-prepare all of the meals in advance for the entire week. You may also schedule each activity down to the very last detail such as what activity you will do, when you will do it, how you will do, how long it will last and any other detail or aspect concerning activity. This level of detailed planning may even include sleeping schedules of what time you go to bed and what time you wake up. It may include every single detail that you can possibly think of that would affect your lifestyle and weight loss efforts. These type of people may also find it helpful to write down and keep track of everything they do.

Some of the benefits of this style of planning are, you leave very little room for error, which may help you maintain control of your weight-loss efforts. It allows you to know exactly what to do and when to do it. It allows you to keep track of your progress. It can also allow you to easily determine what is working and what is not working.

The downside of this level of detailing is that there is no way to plan for everything. Life can sometimes be full of surprises, with this level of detail, any miscalculation can throw your plans into chaos. Most people who are this meticulous and organized do not function very well under chaotic or high stress situations. Another downside of this is that it allows you very little freedom or choice. It can also become very complicated and stressful to maintain this level of organization and detail.

Spontaneous: People who are very spontaneous and not organized, view planning as being restrictive and demoralizing. These people may prefer to go with the flow, improvise and make decisions when they arise. They may wish to make moderate and healthier dietary choices from what is available to them wherever and whenever they're at. They may choose only to eat when they're hungry and not at a specific time. Their activity choices may be the same choosing what they want to do, when they want to do it, according to where they're at and what they have available. These people generally prefer not to write down or keep track of very little detail and instead make adjustments and choices by what feels right.

Some of the benefits of this style may be that it allows for freedom of choice. It can allow for better improvising, which can allow them to compromise and make moderate and healthier choices, even in times when life is not perfect. It can be much simpler and less stressful in certain circumstances.

The downside to this level of planning or lack of planning is that it can be very hard to keep track of what is working and what is not working. The level of commitment to your weight loss efforts can become more sporadic and less consistent, which could undermine your weight-loss efforts. It may become easier to get off course, making your goals that much more difficult to reach.

In-between: Some people may be somewhere in between completely meticulous and completely spontaneous. These people will generally create some kind of balance between the two extremes and utilize aspects from both. This type of person may plan what types of food to eat, but not have a specific meal or day of the week to eat it. They may restrict what they eat, but not when they eat. They might also choose specific attributes or goals to train for, but allow for freedom of time and activity choice. These type of people generally do not record every aspect or detail, but do find some way of keeping track of what works and what does not work.

The benefits of this level of planning can be the same as the benefits from both of the above mentioned level of planning. It can allow you to stay on track and organized, but still allow you freedom of choice and the ability to improvise.

The downside to this level of planning may be none too a few depending on whether you can create a good balance or tend to lean towards one of the extremes or the other.

There is lots of opinions on how and to what extent you should plan, but the bottom line is that you must choose what most suits you and your lifestyle according to what type of person you are. It's your lifestyle and no one else's make your own choices and determine what benefits you the most effectively and efficiently.

Factor in the past, present and future

When designing and planning your weight loss program or lifestyle, you should take into consideration your past, present and future. All of these can help or affect your weight loss efforts. Here's a few sayings that I feel is appropriate at this time. "Fail to learn from your past and you're destined to repeat it." "Those who ignore their present, have no future." "The future is only kind to those who prepare for it." Let's take a look at how your past present and future can help or affect your weight loss efforts.

Past: If there was ever a time in your past that you were not overweight, try to figure out what you were doing differently. Even if you have always been overweight, was there a time that you had weight fluctuations? Try to figure out things in the past that may have worked or not have worked. By analyzing your past you can utilize and incorporate the different aspects that worked into your current program or lifestyle. You can also avoid, eliminate or modify the aspects that did not work. Your past is a valuable source of information that you can utilize for your current situation.

Present: This is one of the most important considerations you will make in your designing and planning. The present is where everything happens. This is where you must determine what you're going to do to lose weight. There is various factors that will affect these decisions. These factors can include but are not limited to: Needs, likes, dislikes, beliefs, goals, ability, financial, access and various other factors that may or may not be unique to each individual. Let's take a closer look at some of these factors and see how they might affect your designing and planning phase.

- Needs: Needs will generally outweigh any other factor, these should generally be considered before anything else. Needs will generally be more important than wants, likes, dislikes, etc. This can also work in your favor if you can turn your weight loss into a need rather than just a want it may become much more achievable. You'd be surprised at what you can do when you have to do it and have no other choice.

- Likes and dislikes: This is also a very important factor affecting your weight loss efforts. If you like a food choice you're more likely to eat it, if you dislike a food choice you're less likely to eat it. If you like an activity choice you're more likely to do it. If you dislike an activity choice you are less likely to do it. Get the picture?

- Beliefs: these can come in the form of, generalized beliefs, conditioned beliefs or religious beliefs. If you believe something will work, it is more likely to be effective. If you believe something will not work, it is less likely to be effective. If you believe something is wrong or immoral it will be counterproductive to your goals.

- Goals: These are what you want and will be the primary reason for designing and planning a program or lifestyle. Your design and plan should be structured to allow you to reach these goals. Goals can include various attributes, skills or aspects including but not limited to: muscle development, leanness, endurance, strength, combat skills, sports skills, work related skills, lifestyle skills and various other aspects or combination of aspects. Your program or lifestyle design and plan should be structured to allow you to reach these goals. You cannot eat and train like a marathon runner to develop massive muscles. You cannot eat and training like a bodybuilder to prepare yourself for a marathon.

- Ability: This refers to your means or actual ability to do something. This must be considered when developing your program or lifestyle. If you are allergic to a certain food you should not include it into your dietary plans. If you cannot run a mile, then you should not plan to run 5 miles for three times a week. You must realistically consider your current abilities when designing, planning or changing your weight loss program or lifestyle.

- Other factors: some of the other factors can include financial, if you cannot afford a gym membership you should not plan to use the gym. Access, if you do not have access to a swimming pool do not design your program or lifestyle around swimming activity. Various other factors that may affect your weight-loss efforts are, once again including but not limited to: family, friends, health concerns, equipment access or availability, age, environment, geographical location, and various other factors, some of which may be completely unique to each individual.

As you can see there is many factors that will affect your weight loss efforts, you should consider all of the factors that may affect you in your weight loss efforts before designing or planning any weight-loss program or lifestyle. These considerations must be taken into account for the present and current situation.

Future: A lot of people fail to consider the future when designing and planning a weight-loss program or lifestyle. They seem to think that they can cut their calories and increase activity until they lose the weight and then they believe they can return to normal. You must remember that what you do to lose the weight, may be what you have to continue to do in order to maintain the weight loss. A good rule of thumb to follow is, when you are designing or planning a dietary or activity change, ask yourself if you can maintain and continue to do or incorporate this change for the rest of your life or for however long you wish to maintain the weight loss. Many things can change including some of the factors that effect your weight loss efforts in the present. You should consider this and be prepared to deal with, modify, customize, improvise and accept any changes the future may bring known or unknown.

I hope you can now see why you must factor in the past, present and future.

Here is another saying that you can ponder. "Learn from the past, live in the present and prepare for the future."

ACTION PHASE

After you've evaluated yourself and your situation, gathered information, designed and planned a preliminary program or lifestyle that is based on realistic information concerning your past, present and future, it is time to take action.

Before you begin

Before you begin you will need to determine your starting point in order to measure progress. Use one or more of the weight evaluation methods, weigh, take measurements and/or take any photos and save or record the results in some way for future reference. By doing this you will be able to monitor your progress more efficiently. Remember, only use what you wish to use that is convenient and simple for you, to ensure that you will actually do it.

Getting started

Don't try to fix everything all at once, utilize patience and moderation. Progress at your own pace that is comfortable and efficient for you. Start with either one of your major concerns and focus on this alone or start working on one or more of your smaller concerns. If you try to tackle everything at once, it will be much more difficult to maintain. Break it down into smaller segments in order to simplify.

What you start with is completely up to you. However, I suggest starting with the major or worst concern you have. The reasons I suggest this is by taking your worst problem first and working on it by itself, can make it much easier to succeed at correcting this problem. Also a lot of people find that once they have corrected their major problem that is enough and the smaller problems are not as much of a concern as they thought. Another reason is when you correct your major concern you will see the biggest results. The last reason is that by correcting your biggest concern, will give you confidence making the smaller concerns much easier to deal with.

Moderate progression

In order to lose weight you must create a calorie deficit, you can do this by decreasing the calories you consume through food, increasing activity or a combination of both. You must realize however, if you create too large of a calorie deficit your body will think that it is starving and fight against you. This is sometimes referred to as the "starvation mode." When your body goes into this mode it will start to store fat, breakdown muscle tissue and slow down your metabolism. When this happens even if you lose weight , the weight will come from muscle and you will be fatter even at a lighter weight.

To prevent the starvation mode you should utilize moderate progression. Slowly incorporate change and gradually allow your body and yourself to adjust to this change. Once you have adjusted you can gradually introduce more change. Continue this moderate progression until you reach your goals. Also keep in mind that the slower you lose the weight the easier it will be, to not only lose the weight but to also maintain this weight loss. As a general guideline there is no minimum weight you should lose. The maximum weight you should lose is no more than 1-2 pounds per week.

The 80% rule

This rule is generally meant to be applied to dietary efforts, but it can be applied to all weight-loss efforts. This rule simply means that you should be strict with your weight-loss efforts 80% of the time this would leave you with 20% of nonrestrictive freedom. Here's what this rule would look like calculated for a weekly basis. There are seven days in a week so multiply 7 x 80 percent which would give you a value of 5.6 days subtract 5.6 from seven would leave you with 1.4 days or just slightly more than one day. (7 x 80% = 5.6) (7 - 5.6 = 1.4) by rounding everything out this would leave you with around six days of weight-loss efforts and one free day.

Simply put you should allow yourself at least one free day a week. Some people refer to this as a cheat day, but in my opinion there is nothing about it that involves cheating. It is actually necessary and important part of your weight loss efforts. The healthiest people almost always follow this rule to some extent or another. Even if you look at people who try to maintain 100% perfection these people although very skinny are very seldom healthy. They generally have very low muscle and low energy, and even though they are skinny they have fairly high body fat percentages. Let's take a closer look at how you can apply this rule to both dietary efforts and activity.

Dietary efforts: No matter how you break this down it comes out to approximately 1 free day a week. Calculating weekly you get 1.4 days a week. If you calculate three meals a day not counting snacks it looks like this 3 meals a day x 7 days a week = 21 meals per week (3 x 7 = 21). 80% of 21 is 16.8 , 21 - 16.8 = 4.2 this would still leave you with a little more than one days worth of meals. If you factor in the snacks or what most fitness trainers recommend of eating six times a day it looks like this 6 x 7 = 42, 42 x 80% = 33.6, 42 - 33.6 = 8.4 leaving you with 8.4 meals a week or just over one days worth of meals. So to simplify simply allow yourself one free day a week that you do not restrict what you eat. Eat whatever you want, just don't go overboard.

By utilizing this method with your dietary efforts not only will it make your efforts easier but it will also keep your body from going into the starvation mode that we talked about earlier. This will allow your metabolism to stay high, allowing you to reach your weight loss goals much more easier, efficiently, effectively and healthier.

Activity efforts: Taking the above weekly calculation we got 1.4 free days a week. So how does this apply to activity? Simple, if you remember the information about recovery that we discussed earlier in this book, you know you should have at least one day of static recovery and one day of active recovery, this would be equal to 20% unrestricted freedom and would follow the 80% rule.

That is how this rule applies to both dietary and activity efforts. Remember, a too restrictive program or lifestyle will be extremely hard to follow and maintain. Apply the 80% rule and give yourself a little bit of freedom and increase your success rate. Everybody needs a little bit of freedom, live free and have fun.

Monitoring progress

To monitor your progress simply use the same evaluation tools or techniques that you used to begin with, and compare the two results. As a general guideline photos should only be taken around every 30 days, any sooner might not show any visible results. The weighing and measurements can be taken once a week. Some people recommend weighing every day, however, it is important to be aware that your weight will naturally fluctuate throughout the week. Some individuals weight fluctuation can be as much as 5 pounds. If you choose to weigh every day you must determine your natural weight fluctuation and factor this in, in order to get an accurate progress evaluation. What ever you choose is fine, just keep it simple and efficient.

Maintenance and beyond

If you have gradually and moderately incorporated change, and made steady moderate progress, then maintenance is simple. Just continue to do what you're doing when you reach your goals. You should now be completely in control of your weight and your life. Simple manipulations of different factors will allow you to make any changes you want to make from now on.

If you want to build more muscle, you may need to do one or combination of the following. Increase resistance training, decrease endurance training, and/or slightly increase calorie intake (preferably from protein).

If you wish to become leaner, you can do one or more of the following. Increase endurance training, change lower rep resistance training to higher rep resistance training, and/or decrease calorie intake (preferably from carbs).

The choices are endless, just remember to keep it simple, efficient, effective and fun.

FINAL SUGGESTIONS

Here are some final suggestions that I hope you will find helpful in your weight-loss effort. Once again these are only suggestions utilize as many or as little of these as you wish or simply ignore them all and find your own way. Your way is the right way.

Dietary suggestions:

- Start with worthless foods that are devoid of any nutritional value.

- Eliminate or substitute healthier foods in place of sugary foods and drinks, highly processed food items, and foods that contain chemicals or ingredients that you don't know what they are, or cannot pronounce.

- Incorporate ways to slow your eating down.

- Slowly reduce the amount of food you eat.

- Eat smaller more frequent meals.
- Eat only when you're actually hungry, but before you become extremely hungry.
- Occupy your time to avoid eating from of boredom.

Activity suggestions:

- Slowly increase the amount or intensity of any activity you currently do.
- Slowly incorporate moderate amounts of activity throughout your day.
- Use your time productively every day.
- Utilize activity that you enjoy for the majority of your activity choices.
- If you wish to conduct specific or specialized training make sure your equipment and exercises is also specific to your goals.
- Always conduct activity in a safe and productive manner.
- Have fun.

Mental training suggestions:

- Utilize deep breathing and mental relaxation periodically throughout your day.

- Utilize visualization to improve weight loss efforts.

- Utilize positive thoughts in order to keep your mindset and attitude positive.

- Utilize mental focus to focus on what you are doing at any particular time.

- Relax, don't worry, be happy, have fun and live life.

BOTTOM LINE

The bottom line is that there is no magic pill, there is no miracle food, there is no superior exercise and there is no mental tricks to make you instantly lose weight. There is only common sense, self-control, effort and determination. There is no one single way of doing anything, there is multiple ways of doing everything, you must experiment and determine what is best for you. Weight loss is not a race or a test, keep it simple and progress at your own pace. Simplify, customize and personalize anything you need to, in order to get the job done.

This is your life and your weight-loss effort, be open to advice but do not blindly follow any of it. Use what you have available to the best of your ability, anywhere, anytime and anyway. Use common sense, follow your heart and your mind, take control, live free, have fun and make the best of the life you have. I know you can succeed because I believe in you, so believe in yourself and nothing will stand in your way.

Good luck and best wishes!

Tim Dutton

Tim Dutton Investigations

C.O.T.A. Training Center

BONUS # 1:

FOOD ADDITIVES AT A GLANCE

Food manufacturers put additives into foods for the purpose of flavor enhancement, filling, preserving, visual enhancement, thickening, nutritional enhancement, volumizing and various other known and unknown reasons. Some of these food additives are considered safe, some are considered unsafe and the safety of some of the additives is unknown, yet food manufacturers continue and are allowed to continue to put these additives in the foods that you consume on an everyday basis.

It is ultimately up to the consumer to determine whether the nutritional value and or taste of a food is worth the risk. However, when consumers read labels they may not be able to even pronounce the word much less determine what it is. So let's take a quick look at some of these additives, In order to give you a better understanding of these additives and allow you to be able to make a more informed choice.

High-risk

These are the additives that has either been proven to be unsafe in the quantities consumed or that have not been properly tested to determine whether they are safe or not. You should avoid these additives because the risk outweighs the value.

ACESULFAME-K

What it is or what its used for: Artificial sweetener.

Products that may contain this additive: Baked goods, chewing gum, gelatin desserts, diet soda, and other artificially sweetened products.

Possible risk: Increased risk of cancer and thyroid problems.

ASPARTAME

What it is or what its used for: Artificial sweetener.

Products that may contain this additive: Diet soda, drink mixes, gelatin desserts, low calorie frozen desserts, sweetener packets and other artificially sweetened products.

Possible risk: Increased risk of cancer, brain tumors, leukemia, lymphoma and breast cancer.

BLUE 1

What it is or what its used for: Artificial Color.

Products that may contain this additive: Beverages, candy and baked goods.

Possible risk: Small increase of cancer risk.

BLUE 2

What it is or what its used for: Artificial color.

Products that may contain this additive: Beverages, candy and pet food.

Possible risk: Studies suggest but do not prove that this additive make cause brain tumors.

BUTYLATED HYDROXYYANISOLE (BHA)

What it is or what its used for: Antioxidant. This additive is used to retard rancidity in fat, oils and oil-containing foods.

Products that may contain this additive: Cereal, chewing gum, potato chips and vegetable oil.

Possible risk: Increase in cancer risk.

CYCLAMATE

What it is or what its used for: Artificial sweetener.

Products that may contain this additive: Diet foods and other artificially sweetened products.

Possible risk: Increases potency of carcinogens. (Carcinogens are cancer causing substances or agents).

GREEN 3

What it is or what its used for: Artificial color.

Products that may contain this additive: Candy and artificially colored beverages.

Possible risk: Possible cause of bladder cancer.

OLESTRA (Olean)

What it is or what its used for: Fat substitute.

Products that may contain this additive: Lay's light chips and Pringles light chips.

Possible risk: Mild to severe diarrhea, loose stools, abdominal cramps, flatulence and other adverse effects.

PARTIALLY HYDROGENATED VEGETABLE OIL, HYDROGENATED VEGETABLE OIL (TRANS FAT)

What it is or what its used for: Fat and oil shortening. This is used to turn fats and oils from liquid states into semi-solid states.

Products that may contain this additive: Stick margarines, crackers, fried restaurant foods, baked goods, icing, microwave popcorn and fast food products.

Possible risk: Heart and artery disease.

POTASSIUM BROMATE

What it is or what its used for: Flour improver. Used to increase the volume and fine crumb structure of bread.

Products that may contain this additive: White flour, bread and rolls.

Possible risk: Increased risk of cancer.

PROPYL GALLATE

What it is or what its used for: Antioxidant preservative. Retards spoilage of fats and oils.

Products that may contain this additive: Vegetable oil, meat products, potato sticks, chicken soup base and chewing gum.

Possible risk: Possible increased risk of cancer.

RED 3

What it is or what its used for: Artificial color.

Products that may contain this additive: Cherries in fruit cocktail, candy and baked goods.

Possible risk: May cause thyroid tumors.

SACCHARIN

What it is or what its used for: Artificial sweetener.

Products that may contain this additive: Diet products, no sugar added products, soft drinks, sweetener packets and other artificially sweetened products.

Possible risk: Increased risk of cancer in bladder, uterus, ovaries, skin, blood vessels and other organs. Also increases potency of other cancer-causing chemicals.

SODIUM NITRITE, SODIUM NITRATE

What it is or what its used for: Preservative, color stabilizer, flavor enhancer. It is used to stabilize the red color in cured meat and also gives characteristic flavor.

Products that may contain this additive: Bacon, ham, frankfurters, hot dogs, sausage, luncheon meats, beef jerky, smoked fish, corned beef and other cured meat products.

Possible risk: Possible increased risk of various cancers.

YELLOW 6

What it is or what its used for: Artificial color.

Products that may contain this additive: Beverages, sausage, baked goods, candy and gelatin.

Possible risk: Tumors of the adrenal gland and kidneys. Also contains small amounts of several carcinogens. May also cause occasional allergic reactions.

Avoid if possible

These are additives that may pose a possible risk and needs to be more properly tested. You should try to avoid these as much as possible and use at your own risk.

BROMINATED VEGETABLE OIL (BVO)

What it is or what its used for: Emulsifier and clouding agent. Used to keep flavor oils in suspension and to give a cloudy appearance to citrus-flavored soft drinks.

Products that may contain this additive: Soft drinks.

Possible risk: This additive leaves small residues in body fat, it is unknown whether these residues pose any risk.

BUTYLATED HYDROXYTOLUENE (BHT)

What it is or what its used for: Antioxidant. Retards rancidity in oils.

Products that may contain this additive: Cereals, chewing gum, potato chips, oils, etc.

Possible risk: Unknown. Tests inconclusive. Increased risk or decreased risk of cancer.

CITRUS RED 2

What it is or what its used for: Artificial color.

Products that may contain this additive: Skin of some Florida oranges only.

Possible risk: Slight increased risk of cancer.

DIACETYL

What it is or what its used for: Butter flavoring.

Products that may contain this additive: Butter, butter-flavored popcorn, margarine, butter-flavored cooking oils and sprays.

Possible risk: Long term exposure causes obstructive lung disease, which can be potentially fatal.

HEPTYL PARABEN

What it is or what its used for: Preservative.

Products that may contain this additive: Beer and non-carbonated soft drinks.

Possible risk: Not tested for long term use, also has not been tested in the presence alcohol, even though it is used in alcohol containing beverages.

RED 40

What it is or what its used for: Artificial color.

Products that may contain this additive: Soda pop, candy, gelatin desserts, pastries, sausage and junk food.

Possible risk: Unknown. Tests were flawed and inconclusive.

QUININE

What it is or what its used for: Flavoring.

Products that may contain this additive: Tonic water, quinine water and bitter lemon.

Possible risk: Slight chance of birth defects. This additive is poorly tested.

Use sparingly

These are additives that are considered safe in small quantities but may pose a risk or promote bad nutrition when large quantities are consumed. You should try to cut back on the products containing these additives and consume them in smaller quantities and less often.

CORN SYRUP

What it is or what its used for: Sweetener and thickener.

Products that may contain this additive: Candy, marshmallows, syrups, snack foods, imitation dairy foods and junk food.

Possible risk: Has no nutritional value just empty calories, can promote weight gain and tooth decay.

DEXTROSE

What it is or what its used for: Sweetener.

Products that may contain this additive: Bread, caramel, soda pop, cookies and various other products.

Possible risk: Empty calories, can promote weight gain and tooth decay.

FRUCTOSE

What it is or what its used for: Sweetener.

Products that may contain this additive: Health drinks, sports drinks, fruit flavored drinks and various other products.

Possible risk: This additive is safe in moderate amounts. However, in large amounts it can increase triglyceride (fat) levels in blood, increasing the risk of heart disease. Consuming large amounts on a regular basis also can affect levels of appetite regulating hormones such as insulin, leptin and ghrelin, thereby increasing the risk of weight gain and obesity.

HIGH-FRUCTOSE CORN SYRUP (HFCS)

What it is or what its used for: Sweetener.

Products that may contain this additive: Soft drinks, junk food and various other processed food and beverage products.

Possible risk: Can promote weight gain and obesity.

HYDROGENATED STARCH HYDROLYSATE (HSH)

What it is or what its used for: Sweetener.

Products that may contain this additive: Diet and reduced calorie foods.

Possible risk: Consuming large amounts of this attitude may cause intestinal gas and diarrhea.

INVERT SUGAR

What it is or what its used for: Sweetener.

Products that may contain this additive: Candy, soft drinks and various other products.

Possible risk: Empty calories, can promote weight gain and tooth decay.

LACTITOL

What it is or what its used for: Sweetener.

Products that may contain this additive: Sugar-free candy, chocolates, baked goods, ice cream and various other sugar-free products.

Possible risk: Large amounts of this additive make calls loose stools or diarrhea.

MALITOL

What it is or what its used for: Sweetener.

Products that may contain this additive: Sugar-free candy, chocolates, jams and various other sugar-free products.

Possible risk: Large amounts of the sedative may have a laxative effect, causing diarrhea.

MANNITOL

What it is or what its used for: Sweetener, duster and various other uses.

Products that may contain this additive: The dust on chewing gum, diet foods and various other low-calorie products.

Possible risk: Consuming large amounts of this additive may have a laxative effect, leading to loose stools and diarrhea.

POLYDEXTROSE

What it is or what its used for: Bulking agent.

Products that may contain this additive: Reduced-calorie salad dressings, baked goods, candy, puddings and frozen desserts.

Possible risk: Consuming large amounts may have a laxative effect.

SALATRIM

What it is or what its used for: Modified fat.

Products that may contain this additive: Baked goods and candy.

Possible risk: Consuming large amounts of this additive can cause stomach cramps and nausea. Very little testing has been done on this additive.

SORBITOL

What it is or what its used for: Sweetener, thickening agent and moisture maintainer.

Products that may contain this additive: Diet drinks, diet foods, candy, shredded coconut and chewing gum.

Possible risk: Consuming large amounts of this additive may have a laxative effect.

SUGAR (SUCROSE)

What it is or what its used for: Sweetener.

Products that may contain this additive: Table sugar and various sweetened products.

Possible risk: Can promote obesity and tooth decay.

TAGATOSE

What it is or what its used for: Sugar substitute.

Products that may contain this additive: Used in place of sugar.

Possible risk: Large amounts may cause nausea.

XYLITOL

What it is or what its used for: Sweetener.

Products that may contain this additive: Sugar-free chewing gum and various other low-calorie products.

Possible risk: Large amounts may cause a laxative effect.

Allergy or sensitivity issues

These are additives that certain people may be sensitive to or may promote light, moderate or high allergic reactions. They should be avoided by certain people who have high sensitivity or are prone to allergic reactions from food and/or beverage products.

ARTIFICIAL AND NATURAL FLAVORING

What it is or what its used for: Flavoring and flavor enhancer.

Products that may contain this additive: Soda pop, candy, cereals, gelatin desserts, fruit juices and various other food and beverage products.

Possible risk: When food labels contain this ingredient it generally means that the real thing has been left out. Companies use various chemicals and they usually keep them a secret. Some of these chemicals may cause a allergic reaction in certain individuals.

CAFFEINE

What it is or what its used for: Stimulant.

Products that may contain this additive: Naturally present in coffee, cocoa, tea, coffee flavored yogurt and frozen desserts. Used as an additive in soft drinks, energy drinks, sports drinks, gum and waters.

Possible risk: This is considered a drug and is mildly addictive, (this is why most companies add it to their products). When suddenly stopped users can experience withdrawal symptoms, similar to withdrawal from other drugs including headaches, irritability, sleepiness and lethargy.

Caffeine can also increase the risk of miscarriages and birth defects and inhibits fetal growth in pregnant women. Therefore, it should be avoided during pregnancy.

Consuming large amounts of caffeine can cause jitters, nervousness, prevent sleeping, affects calcium metabolism and can cause heart palpitations or heart racing.

CARMINE (COCHINEAL EXTRACT)

What it is or what its used for: Artificial color.

Products that may contain this additive: Red, pink or purple candy, yogurt, ice cream, beverages and various other products. This additive is also used in drugs and cosmetics.

Possible risk: Can cause mild to severe allergic reactions such as hives or anaphylactic shock, in some individuals.

CASEIN (SODIUM CASEINATE)

What it is or what its used for: Thickening and whitening agent.

Products that may contain this additive: Ice cream, ice milk, sherbet, coffee creamers some non-dairy and vegetarian foods.

Possible risk: Some people are highly allergic to casein.

HYDROLYZED VEGETABLE PROTEIN (HVP)

What it is or what its used for: Flavor enhancer.

Products that may contain this additive: Instant soups, frankfurters, sauce mixes and beef stew.

Possible risk: HVP contains MSG and may cause adverse reactions in certain individuals.

LACTOSE

What it is or what its used for: Sweetener.

Products that may contain this additive: Naturally present in milk. Used as an additive in Whipped topping mix and breakfast pastries.

Possible risk: Many individuals have trouble digesting lactose and can cause gas and bloating.

MONOSODIUM GLUTAMATE (MSG)

What it is or what its used for: Flavor enhancer.

Products that may contain this additive: Soup, salad dressing, chips, frozen entrees, restaurant and fast food.

Possible risk: Headaches, weakness, wheezing, changes in heart rate, difficulty breathing and burning sensations in back of neck and forearms. Large amounts may destroy nerve cells in the brain.

MYCOPROTEIN (QUORN)

What it is or what its used for: Meat substitute.

Products that may contain this additive: Quorn brand foods.

Possible risk: Vomiting, nausea, diarrhea, hives and anaphylactic reactions.

TRAGACANTH GUM

What it is or what its used for: Thickening agent and stabilizer.

Products that may contain this additive: Beverages, ice cream, frozen pudding, salad dressing, dough, cottage cheese, candy and drink mixes.

Possible risk: Occasional severe allergic reactions.

SODIUM BENZOATE (BENZOIC ACID)

What it is or what its used for: Preservative.

Products that may contain this additive: Fruit juice, carbonated drinks and pickles.

Possible risk: Can cause hives, asthma or other allergic reactions in sensitive individuals.

SULFITES (SULFUR DIOXIDE) (SODIUM BISULFITE)

What it is or what its used for: Preservative and bleach.

Products that may contain this additive: Dried fruit, wine and processed potatoes.

Possible risk: Can cause severe allergic reactions in sensitive individuals, especially in asthmatics.

VANILLIN (ETHYL VANILLIN)

What it is or what its used for: Vanilla substitute.
Products that may contain this additive: Ice cream, baked goods, beverages, chocolate, candy and gelatin desserts.

Possible risk: Certain individuals can be allergic.

YELLOW 5

What it is or what its used for: Artificial color.

Products that may contain this additive: Gelatin desserts, candy, baked goods and pet foods.

Possible risk: Mild allergic reactions, primarily in aspirin-sensitive persons.

Considered safe

These are food additives that are considered or appear to be relatively safe. They are considered to not pose a health risk, therefore, no unnecessary steps need to be taken to avoid these additives. However, you should pay attention to your body, utilize your instincts and make your own choices.

ALGINATE (PROPYLENE GLYCOL ALGINATE)

What it is or what its used for: Thickening agent and foam stabilizer.

Products that may contain this additive: Ice cream, cheese, candy, yogurt and beer.

Possible risk: Appears to be safe.

ALPHA TOCOPHEROL (VITAMIN E)

What it is or what its used for: Antioxidant and nutrient.

Products that may contain this additive: Vegetable oils, breakfast cereals and beverages.

Possible risk: Appears to be safe.

ASCORBIC ACID (VITAMIN C) (SODIUM ASCORBATE)

What it is or what its used for: Antioxidant, nutrient and color stabilizer.

Products that may contain this additive: Cereals, fruit drinks and cured meats.

Possible risk: Appears to be safe.

BETA-CAROTENE

What it is or what its used for: Coloring and nutrient.

Products that may contain this additive: Margarine, shortening, non-dairy whiteners, beverages, breakfast cereals and supplements.

Possible risk: Appears to be safe.

CALCIUM or SODIUM PROPIONATE

What it is or what its used for: Preservative.

Products that may contain this additive: Bread, rolls, pies and cakes.

Possible risk: Appears to be safe.

CALCIUM or SODIUM STEAROYL LACTYLATE (CALCIUM or SODIUM STEAROYL FUMARATE)

What it is or what its used for: Dough conditioner and whipping agent.

Products that may contain this additive: Bread dough, cake fillings, artificial whipped cream and processed egg whites.

Possible risk: Appears to be safe.

CARRAGEENAN

What it is or what its used for: Thickening, gelling and stabilizing agent.

Products that may contain this additive: Ice cream, jelly, chocolate milk, infant formula and cottage cheese.

Possible risk: Appears to be safe.

CITRIC ACID (SODIUM CITRATE)

What it is or what its used for: Acid, flavoring and chelating agent.

Products that may contain this additive: Ice cream, sherbet, fruit drinks, candy, carbonated beverages and instant potatoes.

Possible risk: Appears to be safe.

DIACYLGLYCEROL

What it is or what its used for: Emulsifier.

Products that may contain this additive: Cooking oil.

Possible risk: Appears to be safe.

EDTA

What it is or what its used for: Chelating agent.

Products that may contain this additive: Salad dressing, margarine, sandwich spreads, mayonnaise, processed fruits, processed vegetables, canned shellfish and soft drinks.

Possible risk: Appears to be safe.

ERYTHORBIC ACID

What it is or what its used for: Antioxidant and color stabilizer.

Products that may contain this additive: Cured meats.

Possible risk: Appears to be safe.

FERROUS GLUCONATE

What it is or what its used for: Coloring and nutrient.

Products that may contain this additive: Black olives.

Possible risk: Appears to be safe.

FUMARIC ACID

What it is or what its used for: Tartness agent.

Products that may contain this additive: Powdered drinks, pudding, pie fillings and gelatin desserts.

Possible risk: Appears to be safe.

GELATINE

What it is or what its used for: Thickening and gelling agent.

Products that may contain this additive: Powdered dessert mixes, marshmallows, yogurt, ice cream, cheese spreads and beverages.

Possible risk: Appears to be safe.

GLYCERIN (GLYCEROL)

What it is or what its used for: Maintains water content.

Products that may contain this additive: Candy, fudge and baked goods.

Possible risk: Appears to be safe.

GUMS (ARABIC, FURCELLERAN, GHATTI, GUAR, KARAYA, LOCUST BEAN, and XANTHAN)

What it is or what its used for: Thickening agents and stabilizers.

Products that may contain this additive: Beverages, ice cream, frozen pudding, salad dressing, dough, cottage cheese, candy and drink mixes.

Possible risk: Appears to be safe.

HIGH MALTOSE CORN SYRUP

What it is or what its used for: Improve shelf life, inhibits bacterial growth, fermentation and various other purposes.

Products that may contain this additive: Candy, baked goods and beer.

Possible risk: Appears to be safe.

INULIN

What it is or what its used for: Fat substitute.

Products that may contain this additive: Margarine, baked goods, fillings, dairy foods, frozen desserts and salad dressing.

Possible risk: Appears to be safe.

LACTIC ACID

What it is or what its used for: Controls acidity.

Products that may contain this additive: Spanish olives, cheese, frozen desserts and carbonated beverages.

Possible risk: Appears to be safe.

LECITHIN

What it is or what its used for: Emulsifier and antioxidant.

Products that may contain this additive: Baked goods, margarine, chocolate and ice cream.

Possible risk: Appears to be safe.

MALTODEXTRIN

What it is or what its used for: Dietary fiber simulator.

Products that may contain this additive: Numerous processed foods.

Possible risk: Appears to be safe.

MONO-DIGLYCERIDES and DIGLYCERIDES

What it is or what its used for: Emulsifier.

Products that may contain this additive: Baked goods, margarine, candy and peanut butter.

Possible risk: Appears to be safe.

NEOTAME

What it is or what its used for: Artificial sweetener.

Products that may contain this additive: Diet soft drinks and other diet food or beverage products.

Possible risk: Appears to be safe.

OAT FIBER (WHEAT FIBER)

What it is or what its used for: Isolated fiber.

Products that may contain this additive: Cereal, crackers, bread and muffins.

Possible risk: Appears to be safe.

OLIGOFRUCTOSE

What it is or what its used for: Bulking agent, emulsifier and sweetener prebiotic.

Products that may contain this additive: Frozen desserts, cookies, energy bars and granola bars.

Possible risk: Appears to be safe.

PHOSPHORIC ACID (PHOSPHATES)

What it is or what its used for: Acidulant, chelating agent, buffer, emulsifier, nutrient and discoloration inhibitor.

Products that may contain this additive: Baked goods, cheese, powdered foods, cured meat, soda pop, breakfast cereals and dehydrated potatoes.

Possible risk: Appears to be safe.

PHYTOSTEROLS and PHYTOSTANOLS (PLANT STEROLS or STANOLS)

What it is or what its used for: Cholesterol-lowering additive.

Products that may contain this additive: Margarine, fruit juice, bread and dietary supplements.

Possible risk: Appears to be safe.

POLYSORBATE 60

What it is or what its used for: Emulsifier.

Products that may contain this additive: Baked goods, frozen desserts and imitation cream.

Possible risk: Appears to be safe.

SODIUM CARBOXYMETHYL-CELLULOSE (CMC)

What it is or what its used for: Thickening agent, stabilizing agent and prevents sugar from crystallizing.

Products that may contain this additive: Ice cream, beer, pie fillings, icings, diet foods and candy.

Possible risk: Appears to be safe.

SORBIC ACID (POTASSIUM SORBATE)

What it is or what its used for: Prevents growth of mold.

Products that may contain this additive: Cheese, syrup, jelly, cake, wine and dried fruits.

Possible risk: Appears to be safe.

SORBITAN MONOSTEARATE

What it is or what its used for: Emulsifier.

Products that may contain this additive: Cakes, candy, frozen pudding and icing.

Possible risk: Appears to be safe.

STARCH

What it is or what its used for: Thickening agent.

Products that may contain this additive: Soup, gravy and frozen foods.

Possible risk: Appears to be safe.

STARCH, MODIFIED (FOOD-STARCH, MODIFIED)

What it is or what its used for: Thickening agent.

Products that may contain this additive: Soup, gravy and frozen foods.

Possible risk: Appears to be safe.

SUCRALOSE

What it is or what its used for: Artificial sweetener.

Products that may contain this additive: No-sugar added baked goods, frozen desserts, ice cream, soft drinks and tabletop sweetener (Splenda).

Possible risk: Appears to be safe.

THAIMAN MONONITRATE (VITAMIN B1)

What it is or what its used for: Nutrient.

Products that may contain this additive: Numerous food and beverage products.

Possible risk: Appears to be safe.

TRIACETIN (GLYCEROL TRIACETATE)

What it is or what its used for: Wetting agent.

Products that may contain this additive: Various beverage products.

Possible risk: Appears to be safe.

Closing statement

As you can see there are numerous additives being placed in our food and beverage products. We have no ideal of how many or how much chemicals are being put into our bodies on a daily basis. Some of these additives are claimed to be natural, but common sense tells us when you add an ingredient natural or not into a product that it does not naturally occur in, then this is no longer natural. Our bodies do not know what to do with some of these chemicals so even the chemicals that are claimed to be safe requires our bodies to do extra work in order to process and filter these chemicals through our bodies.

The primary reason companies place additives into our foods is simply to make more money. If they add thickeners or fillers they can sell less product for more money. If they add enhancers it can make the product more pleasing and cause consumers to buy more of this product. The primary reason that government agencies allow companies to put additives into food products is also because of money and also government agencies do not have the budget or organizational skills to regulate every food product distributor, processor and server.

The rise in obesity and other health related issues and diseases can be directly linked to the timeline of when additives started to be placed in food.

As consumers we have to realize that the more natural a food is with less additives the healthier it will be. We also have to realize that we, as consumers are ultimately in control. If consumers stopped purchasing foods that had additives placed in them, then the companies would be forced to remove these additives. Use your own judgment and common sense. Be safe and be well.

Tim Dutton

Tim Dutton investigations

C.O.T.A. Training Center

BONUS # 2:

WEIGHT LOSS FUN: Calorie Burning Games and Activity Ideas

Weight loss does not have to be something boring or excruciating, that you have to force yourself to do. Weight loss efforts can and should be simple and fun. Here is some game and activity ideas that can help you make your weight loss efforts a little more enjoyable. Some of these ideas are new, some are old but all will burn calories and help to enhance your weight loss efforts.

Dodge ball

Comment: This is a fun game for all ages. You can play with two players or multiple players. It seems to be the most fun when you have two teams of 3-10 players. If you have less than six total players or an odd number of players you can play free for all or last man standing.

Description: The goal is to throw a ball, when you have one, at your opponent or opponents trying to hit them with the ball. If you are the one being thrown at your goal is to either catch or dodge the ball. If a person is hit with a ball they are considered “out”. If a person catches the ball the person that through it is considered “out”. There is generally barriers such as walls, fences, etc. in place to stop the balls and prevent having to chase after them. There is also generally boundaries set for each player or team, forcing them to throw the ball from a certain distance once the other player or team crosses the boundary.

Options: The barriers are optional, without barriers you simply will have to chase after the balls. If you’re playing with a mixture of children and adults, make sure to go easy on the children and have separate rules to make it fair. You can also choose to have 2-3 children equal one player, all must be “tagged” before any of them is considered “out”. This will all depend on age, size and skill level of each child.

Tag/freeze tag

Comment: This is usually considered a child’s game, however, with a little imagination and modification, it can be a fun and valuable calorie burning activity for adults too. This game can be played with two or more people. It can be played utilizing teams or a free for all.

Description: During tag one player or a team of players is designated as “It”. Whoever is “It” must try to tag other players. When someone is tagged they are either out of the game or become "It".

During freeze tag instead of the person tagged being out or becoming "IT", they instead are frozen and must remain in the position that they were tagged in for a specified amount of time.

Both tag and freeze tag generally utilize boundaries that limit's the space or area that can be used for the play area. Both also generally use certain spots or objects that are designated as bases or safe zones. These areas can only be utilized one person at a time and can only be used for a limited amount of time.

Options: Instead of utilizing safe zones you could utilize exercises where someone can not be tagged as long as they are doing a certain type of exercise. You can also utilize exercise in place of freezing, instead of being frozen the person tagged must perform a certain amount of reps of a specific exercise.

Touch/flag/tackle football

Comment: This is another very fun game it can be played rough or toned down to suit your needs. It can be played with two or more players. It is generally played with two teams of players. Contrary to popular belief a large area is not required. Football can be modified and played in surprisingly small areas.

Description: The goal of football is for two teams to compete against each other trying to score touchdowns while preventing the other team from doing the same by touching, pulling a flag or tackling the person that has the ball. Each team generally gets four tries or plays referred to as “downs”, in order to try to score a touchdown. There is also generally first downs awarded after the ball has been moved forward a certain distance which will be determined by the over all playing distance. Generally there is one forward pass allowed per play and unlimited lateral tosses. Football is generally played for a time limit or until one team reaches a specified score.

The only difference in touch football is that instead of tackling the person with the ball, you instead touch or tag them. The area that you can touch or tag is generally a certain spot either on the back or on the lower body.

The difference in flag football is that instead of tackling or touching, each player wears a cloth material, generally placed in the back pocket or in the back of their waistband. To stop the player with the ball the cloth material or “flag” must be pulled out.

Options: Everything is optional. You could limit first downs or do away with them completely depending on the playing area you have available. You can also modify this game completely, and make it more nonstop by doing away with the downs. Each team would simply run for the goal if tackled they would throw the ball up in the air, where it would be scrambled for by every player. If a touchdown is scored the players line up while the ball is thrown as far as it can be thrown and the players must race to get possession of the ball. During play you could allow players to throw the ball to teammates who are only behind them or in front of them or in any direction you choose. This could also be played as a free-for-all instead of having teams.

Exploration hikes/walks

Comment: Hiking and walking are great low intensity calorie burning activities. By adding the exploration element you can not only add a change to keep them interesting, but you can also increase your attention, focus and awareness. This can be done by yourself or with a group. Children especially find this fun.

Description: Add a different element to your normal walk or hike by trying to see or find as many new things as possible.

Options: If you know the area that you will be hiking or walking, you could turn it into a "scavenger hunt", by making a list of items that must be found or seen before you end your walk or hike. To add intensity and a competitive element for more than one person you could turn it into a race where the first person who finds all the items on the list and returns, wins. You could also utilize this with running or jogging instead of hiking or walking, which would increase the intensity and calorie burning effect.

Extreme Simon says

Comment: This could be a light, low intensity workout or an extremely high intensity activity, depending on the competitiveness of the participants. Two or more people can participate in this activity.

Description: This is similar to regular Simon says, the difference is that you will be utilizing exercises or other calorie burning activities and movements. Pick someone to be "Simon", this person will lead the activity, by saying "do this" or "Simon says do this". The participants should only do the activity when it is preceded by "Simon says". When someone fails to do an activity or does an activity that was not preceded by "Simon says", then that person is either out of the game or must do extra reps of an exercise or activity. Game play can continue for a specified amount of time or until there is only one person left.

Options: You can utilize any exercises or activities you choose including but not limited to calisthenics, yoga, Pilates, sprints, resistance training, etc. You can also add a different element to the game play by allowing any person who successfully completes one of the Simon says exercises to challenge Simon with that exercise. The challenger and the current Simon would face off and compete in that particular exercise, the winner would either remain or become "Simon" until he loses a challenge.

Follow the leader

Comment: This can be utilized with any activity or exercise, but it seems to be especially fun when utilizing Parkour or Free-running. It can be used with two or more people.

Description: One person is designated as the leader. Just as the name implies everyone else must follow the leader, doing exactly what he or she does trying to copy it exactly as it is done. Leaders can be rotated as frequently or infrequently as you choose. This continues for a specified amount of time or until the activity is no longer possible to do.

Options: Instead of copying each person exactly you can have each person do what the person in front of them did and then add something new of their own. You would continue to rotate through each person with each person adding something new until someone was no longer capable of completing the required tasks.

Playing card circuit

Comment: This is a very simple way to add variety to your exercises or current program. You can do this by yourself or with a group.

Description: Shuffle a deck of playing cards, designate each suit as a specific exercise. (Example: hearts = push-ups, spades = squats, diamonds = pull-ups, clubs = sit-ups). Deal a card, the suit will represent what exercise you will do, the number will represent the reps or how many times you will do that exercise. The face cards Jack, Queen, King and Ace can be considered a minimum of 10 reps. Continue dealing cards and doing the specified exercise for the specified number of times until you have went through the entire deck. You can re-shuffle and go through the deck as many or as little times as you choose.

Options: The suits can each represent any exercise or activity you choose. The face cards can either represent 10 reps of the exercise for their suit or they can represent a completely different exercise. Joker cards can be left in the deck and can represent a wildcard, where you would do any exercise you chose for any number of reps. The Joker cards could also be utilized for extra rest periods when needed. In order to add intensity go through the deck doing each exercise as quickly as possible and resting only as needed.

Roll of the dice

Comment: This is another way to add variety and randomness to your exercises or current program. This can be done alone or with as many people as you choose.

Description: The numbers on the dice represents the reps or number of times you will perform an exercise. Simply call out an exercise roll the dice and do that exercise for the number of reps that the dice shows. You can utilize one dice or as many dice as you choose. The more dice you utilize the more possible reps you will be required to do.

Options: Instead of the numbers on the dice representing reps, you can have them represent specific exercises. You would predetermine the number of reps you perform such as 5, 10, 15, 20, etc., then designate each rolled number of the dice to represent a specific exercise such as 1 = push-ups, 2 = squats, 3 = pull-ups,
4 = crunches, etc. You would roll the dice and do that exercise for the predetermined number of reps. You can utilize as many dice as you choose, one dice will allow you to do 6 exercises, two dice would allow you to do 11 exercises, etc. (It is important to note that when you use more than one dice, you will not roll a one, even if both dice fall on one, it adds up to two. So keep this in mind when planning this activity).

Catch the bomb

Comment: This is a simple game that can allow you to develop eye hand coordination while burning a few extra calories. You can do it alone or with as many people as you choose.

Description: Choose a ball of any size and type as long as it will not cause serious injury. Throw the ball straight up into the air anyway you can as high as possible. If playing alone try to catch the ball and continue throwing it straight up and re-catching it. If playing with more people, one person will throw, the others will try to catch it. If someone drops the ball they are either out or must perform extra exercise or activity. This game can continue for as long as you wish or until everyone has dropped the ball accept one person, who wins.

Options: Add challenge and intensity by utilizing a weighted medicine ball. By utilizing a medicine ball it will add an element of resistance training and will develop explosive strength for the entire body.

Hot potato

Comment: This is another simple game that can not only allow you to burn extra calories, but also allow you to develop coordination, agility, explosive strength and other fitness attributes. This can be played by two or more people.

Description: If two people are playing stand facing each other. If more than two people are playing stand in a circle equal distances apart. The exact distance will be determined by size and weight of the ball, strength and skill of the player, space available and also personal choice. With two people simply throw the ball back and forth as fast as you can as though it was hot and cannot be touched. With more than two people simply throw the ball to the next person going in a clockwise direction, again as fast as you can. When someone drops the ball they are out. Play continues until only one person is left who has not dropped the ball.

Options: When throwing the ball in a clockwise direction someone can yell switch, in which case whoever is holding the ball at the time would immediately switch directions and the ball would start being thrown in a counterclockwise direction. You can also utilize random throws where you would throw it to anyone you chose, this would require everyone to pay attention and be on their toes. To add intensity and a resistance element you can utilize medicine balls or sandbags.

Annie-over

Comment: My mom came up with this one in order to keep my nieces and nephews entertained. It is fun for all ages, it can be played with as little as two people or as many as you choose. It's the most fun with at least eight or more people. It can also be called "over and around". It combines elements of catch, tag and if you choose dodge ball.

Description: You need some type of structure that will block the view and prevent each team from seeing each other, and to throw a ball over. The structure can be anything you have available including but not limited to a house, a barn, a wall, a shed, a semi trailer, etc. Separate players into two teams, each team should get on opposite sides of the chosen structure. Game play involves throwing a ball of any size or type over the structure. The ball can be thrown completely over the structure or thrown lightly so that it rolls down the other side. The team on the opposite side tries to watch for the ball and tries to catch it. If the ball is not caught, it is simply picked up and thrown back over, you can utilize strategy by waiting a little while before throwing the ball back over. If the ball is caught the entire team runs around the structure in any direction they choose, they can all go in the same direction or in separate directions. The person who caught the ball tries to tag a member from the other team. By having the entire team run around the structure, this can cause confusion and players from the other team must focus to find out who has the ball, before it's too late. If someone is tagged they are either out of the game or they must switch teams. If the players reach the other side of the structure, they are safe and can not be tagged. Play continues until there is no players left on one team.

Options: Instead of tagging a person, you could throw the ball at them, adding an element of dodge ball, the same catching rules in dodge ball applies here as well. Make sure that the ball is of the type that is safe enough that it will not cause injury upon impact. The players that have been tagged out can also still participate. While standing on the side of the structure if their original team drops the ball the tagged out person can stomp their feet making the other team think that the original team caught the ball and is now coming around to tag them, this could cause the opposing team to miss the ball. Tagged out players can also make noise to cover up the sound when their original team is actually coming around to tag someone.

Improvised obstacle course

Comment: This is a very good way to utilize what you have available, to create a fun training and conditioning workout. You can do it by yourself or with as many people as you choose.

Description: Simply find an area that is available to you that has various different objects or structures. This area can be urban or rural and the obstacles can be anything that is available including but not limited to tables, walls, fences, trees, swimming pools, creeks, rocks, monkey bars, benches, bushes, mud puddles, or anything else, it is limited only to your imagination. Determine the path you will take to overcome these obstacles. Run through the chosen path, overcoming obstacles as efficiently, as fast and as safe as you can.

Options: You can do this as simply as a "see if you can do it" type of activity, a race were you compete against someone else, first one through wins, or a timed event where you try to beat someone else's time or your own time as you improve. The course can be as short or as long as you choose. If you live in town it can be contained in your backyard or involve your neighborhood. If you live in the country it can involve one field or your entire acreages. Just utilize common sense and remember no trespassing and no property damage, respect other people's rights, privacy and property.

Cuff the fugitive

Comment: This can be utilized by anyone who wishes, but it is especially beneficial to people who may be required to apprehend someone such as law enforcement officers, bounty hunters, security officers or anyone else who may have to chase and handcuff someone within their chosen profession. This can be a fun way to develop necessary skills. It can be done by two or more people.

Description: This should be kept as realistic as possible while utilizing padding and safety precautions as necessary to prevent injury. One person will be the fugitive, another person will be the one that chases and cuffs. The fugitive should run in any direction they choose and try to escape. The chaser should chase the fugitive and try to get him off balance and onto the ground and handcuff him as quickly and safely as possible.

Options: You can utilize vehicles or structures as starting points. You can utilize obstacles such as fences or walls. You can utilize anything you choose to make it realistic for your personal and needed skill development.

100's

Comment: This is a modification of the basketball game called "H-O-R-S-E". Keep in mind that you can improvise and that you can play this even if you do not have a basketball and goal, just substitute them with something else such as a trash can and a wadded up piece of paper. This can be played with two or more people.

Description: This is played just like H-O-R-S-E except instead of spelling out the word H-O-R-S-E when you miss a shot, you instead do a certain number of reps of any chosen exercise. The first shooter will pick a spot to shoot from and shoot. If he makes it the next player must make the same shot from the same spot. If he makes it, play continues through each player. If the shot is missed that person must perform a certain number of reps of the chosen exercise. Play continues until the total reps of the exercise reaches 100. Once a person reaches 100 reps that person is out of the game.

Options: The reps you choose to utilize can be any number 5, 10, 20, etc. as long as they will total 100. You can alternate who picks each shot, or you can simply continue to pick the shot until you miss.

Hand-to-hand/weapons sparring

Comment: This is very useful for people who are training in or may be required to use self defense. It is a very fun means of burning a tremendous amount of calories, while at the same time developing useful self-defense skills. Two or more people can participate in this activity.

Description: Two opponents square off against each other and spar, trying to score a hit or a submission from their opponent, utilizing kicks, punches, throws, grabs, holds, locks or any other empty hand techniques. Safety equipment and procedures should be utilized to prevent injury.
Weapons sparring is the same except that you're allowed to utilize padded weapons or some other safe form of weapon including but not limited to

paintball guns, padded swords, padded sticks, rubber knives and various other types of safe practice weapons.

Options: You can utilize a contained area or as large a area as you choose. You can spar one-on-one or you can pit one against multiple opponents. You should make this as realistic as possible utilizing various scenarios, while still maintaining safety precautions to avoid injuries.

I hope you find these activities and games fun, enjoyable and beneficial. Remember that these are not the only things available to you. These are simply some examples to make you think and start to utilize your own imagination. If you enjoy an activity then include it within your weight loss or fitness program. If you do not enjoy an activity then either do away with it, change it or modify it so that you do enjoy it. You're in charge of what you do for weight loss and fitness, so make sure that you include beneficial and effective exercises and techniques that you completely enjoy and have fun doing. Have fun, be safe, be effective and utilize what you have available to the best of your ability. Good luck and best wishes.

Tim Dutton
Tim Dutton investigations
C.O.T.A. Training Center

BONUS # 3:

SUPER CHARGE WEIGHT LOSS WITH STAGGERED CALORIES

When you drop your calories to a certain point for prolonged periods of time not only will it be hard to maintain this calorie drop, but your body will also go into starvation mode. When your body goes into starvation mode your metabolism will lower causing you to burn less calories, your body will start to burn calories from muscle and will try to store and conserve the fat. So by dropping calories for prolonged periods of time it can make your weight loss efforts much more difficult and even counterproductive.

There is a method that will not only make it easier to stick with and maintain but also prevent your body from going into starvation mode. This method is known as staggered calories, by utilizing staggered calories, you let your body know that it is not starving and it is also much less restrictive allowing you to maintain your efforts much easier and for longer periods of time. This method also allows you to lose weight much quicker than standard calorie reduction improving your success rate and allowing you to reach your goals sooner. You do not even have to count calories in order to utilize this method. So let's take a look at how the staggered calories method works.

Weekly example

Day 1: Very light day. Consume calories consisting of healthy foods such as fruits, vegetables and lean proteins. Eat small portions periodically throughout the day only when hungry, and eat just enough to subdue the hunger and get adequate nutrition.

Day 2: Moderate day. Eat slightly less than your maintenance needs or what you would normally eat.

Day 3: Normal day. Eat normally or what's required to maintain your weight.

Day 4: Optional. Either have a moderate day or a light day your choice.

Day 5: Moderate day.

Day 6: Very light day.

Day 7: Free day. Slightly higher calorie day. Don't go too extreme, but do allow yourself to eat some of the items you have been avoiding. Don't worry about proper nutrition just simply give yourself a little bit of freedom and enjoy your meals.

If you are counting calories, a very light day would be a calorie reduction or deficit of 500 or more calories below maintenance. A moderate day would be 100-300 calorie deficit. A normal day would be your maintenance level of calories. A free day would be your choice but should be at least 200 calories above your maintenance level.

Personal choice

The above is only an example any combination will work, just make sure that it suits your needs and you are capable of sticking to it. You can start slow with one or two lighter days and slowly reduce food for certain days until you find the combination that gives you the results you want. It is a personal choice you can alternate between light and moderate or moderate and normal or light and normal or any other combination you choose. The only suggestion I make is to make sure you allow yourself one free day a week, this keeps your metabolism raised and also makes dieting much more manageable to stick with. You're in charge, do it the way you want to do it, make the choices for you and what benefits you most efficiently and effectively. Good luck and best wishes.

Tim Dutton

Tim Dutton investigations

C.O.T.A. Training Center

www.ingramcontent.com/pod-product-compliance
Lightning Source LLC
Chambersburg PA
CBHW051345290326
41933CB00042B/3151
9780984083909